the
anatomy
workbook

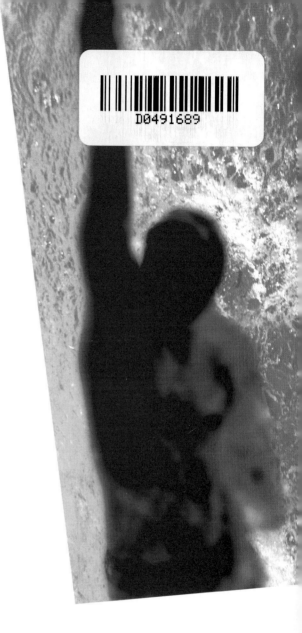

For Butterworth-Heinemann:

Commissioning Editor: Heidi Allen
Project Development Manager: Robert Edwards
Project Manager: Gail Wright
Design Direction: George Ajayi
Cartoonist: Peter Ives

www.fleshandbones.com

The international community for medical students and instructors. Have you joined?

For students

- Free MCQs to test your knowledge
- Online support and revision help for your favourite textbooks
- Student reviews of the books on your reading lists
- Download clinical rotation survival guides
- Win great prizes in our games and competitions

The great online resource for everybody involved in medical education

For instructors

- Download free images and buy others from our constantly growing image bank
- Preview sample chapters from new textbooks
- Request inspection copies
- Browse our reading rooms for the latest information on new books and electronic products
- Secure online ordering with prompt delivery, as well as full contact details to order by phone, fax or post

Log on and register FREE today

fleshandbones.com
– an online resource for medical instructors and students

fleshandbones.com

the anatomy workbook

Stuart Porter BSc(Hons) GradDipPhys
MCSP SRP CertMHS

*Lecturer in Physiotherapy, School of Health Care Professions,
University of Salford, Manchester; Honorary Research Fellow,
Wrightington, Wigan and Leigh NHS Trust, Wigan, UK*

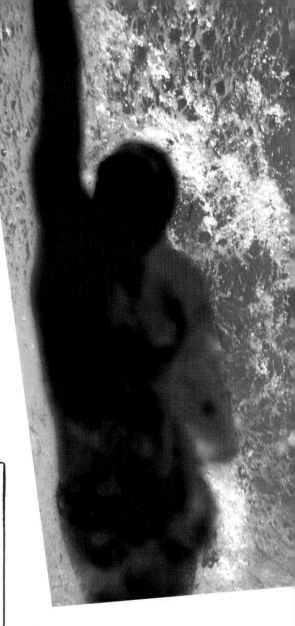

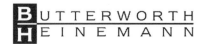

BUTTERWORTH
HEINEMANN

BUTTERWORTH-HEINEMANN
An imprint of Elsevier Limited

First published 2002
Reprinted 2004

ISBN 0 7506 5455 4

British Library Cataloguing in Publication Data
A catalogue record for this book is available from the British
Library

Library of Congress Cataloging in Publication Data
A catalog record for this book is available from the Library of
Congress

Note
Medical knowledge is constantly changing. As new
information becomes available, changes in treatment,
procedures, equipment and the use of drugs become necessary.
The author and the publishers have taken care to ensure that
the information given in this text is accurate and up to date.
However, readers are strongly advised to confirm that the
information, especially with regard to drug usage, complies
with the latest legislation and standards of practice.

your source for books,
journals and multimedia
in the health sciences
www.elsevierhealth.com

The
publisher's
policy is to use
**paper manufactured
from sustainable forests**

Printed in the UK by Martins the Printers Ltd

contents

about the author

I graduated from Manchester Royal Infirmary School of Physiotherapy in 1987 and later obtained a BSc(Hons) degree in Health Studies from Salford University. Initially, I went to work at Wrightington Hospital near Wigan, where I was to specialise eventually in Rheumatology and Orthopaedics. I commenced lecturing in January 1997 and found that I loved it. I worked at Ormskirk District General Hospital as Senior 1 in Orthopaedics and since September 1998 I have been lecturing full-time at the University of Salford. I took students for most of my career in the clinical field and found this to be the most rewarding part of my job. I still work clinically at Wrightington and Ormskirk Hospitals. I am Cyriax trained and for three years I was the physiotherapist to the England women's football team. (My claim to fame is that I am the only *man* to ever be sent off in a *women's* international football match.) I am currently studying for a PhD in exercise compliance in ankylosing spondylitis. My hobbies include photography, amateur astronomy, science fiction (the original Star Trek) and horror films, and I was Wham's greatest fan. I now live with my wife and three girls.

acknowledgements

We rarely pause to thank the people that matter. This is the best chance I will get, so I will take a little of your time to recognise the people that have made a difference in my life, and to whom I owe it all.

To Heidi and Robert at Butterworth-Heinemann, and to Nigel Palastanga, Derek Field and Roger Soames for permission to reproduce figures from their book *Anatomy and Human Movement. Structure and Function*, 4th edn, 2002, published by Butterworth-Heinemann.

To my parents, Brian and Winifred, for believing in me, to Jessica (senior) and Lynn, to Mark for 30 years of friendship. To my students past and future, from whom I learn so much.

To Alison, Claire and Jessica for the fun ahead.

Most of all to Sue – for never giving up, for having faith in me and for the other words that fail me here – you know why.

foreword

Anatomy is often a daunting subject to undergraduate students; it need not be so.

For many years students have yearned for a study guide which covers anatomy in the appropriate depth and detail for their degree courses, but also one which puts the important facts across clearly and succinctly in a form which aids their ongoing study and revision. Although directed at a high academic level and dealing with serious subject matter, *The Anatomy Workbook* helps the student by making the study of anatomy simple, clear and humorous. The subject material is therefore extremely easy to remember as a result – a bonus at examination time.

The format of *The Anatomy Workbook* will appeal to students who want a well laid out study guide to use alongside their academic studies, and the self-directed study projects give scope for more advanced study once the basics have been grasped. Each chapter is a self-contained study unit in its own right, which has clearly set out learning outcomes, diagrams and other useful tips. *The Anatomy Workbook* is a useful study companion to *Anatomy and Human Movement*.

Nigel Palastanga

INTRODUCTION

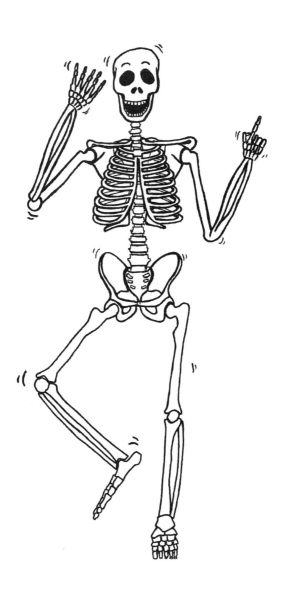

OK so you want to learn anatomy, maybe you need to learn it as part of your undergraduate course, maybe you are about to commence university and want a head start. Maybe you need a quick revision guide as those exams get ever closer. In any event this book should act as a useful study guide. It contains plenty of pretty pictures which students have found useful in the past and silly rhymes and so on to help you get to grip on the important aspects of this huge subject.

THE DESIGN OF THE BOOK

The chapters follow this formula:

JUDGEMENT PAGE
THE JUDGE ASKS YOU WHETHER YOU HAVE ACHIEVED THE CHAPTER'S LEARNING OUTCOMES OR NOT.

THE MAIN TEXT – PLENTY OF SPACES FOR YOUR OWN NOTES AND SELF DIRECTED STUDY PROJECTS.

LEARNING OUTCOMES PAGE
THIS TELLS YOU WHAT I WANT YOU TO GET OUT OF EACH CHAPTER.

COVER PAGE

In the workbook I use friendly language, jokes, rhymes, etc. I do this to make learning easier and more fun. Remember not to write in this style at exam time or in your assignments. I hope that the workbook makes your academic life a little easier.

Some answers to the self-directed study projects appear after the relevant project in the book (the remainder can be obtained from anatomy text books) and there is a reference list in order that you can look deeper into the subject.

ABOUT THE WORKBOOK

This workbook should give you a clear study guide about the important points in anatomy. This can be daunting the first time you open an anatomy textbook. Study and revision needs a structure if it is to be productive – now you have a framework to build your revision upon. After several months as a student, my files were a total mess, this is my attempt to put information together in an organised way to make life as smooth as possible for you – ah what a guy. References are included within the text but only when they serve to link clinical findings to your knowledge of anatomy to illustrate how anatomy cannot be separated from clinical practice.

People in the work book to help you study

The projects that you will need to complete as self-directed study are highlighted by this symbol ...

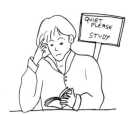

PROFESSOR'S TIP OF THE DAY

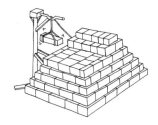

This guy appears every now and again to offer you some wise information.

The stressed out student appears from time to time to help you remember the silly rhymes and word games that you will find useful.

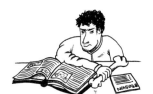

The judge appears at the end of each chapter to assess whether you have achieved the learning outcomes that were set.

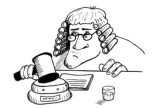

AN INTRODUCTION TO ANATOMY

Think of the workbook as a foundation to build your studies upon.

WHAT THIS WORKBOOK IS

- ☞ This is not another anatomy textbook – there are plenty of those around already. As soon as you get this book, start working through it, studying the text and filling in the blanks and self-directed study sections.
- ☞ It is in the form of a 'Fill in the blanks' interactive workbook and it has enough spaces for you to add your own notes.
- ☞ At the end of the book there is a checklist that will not mean much to you at first but it is designed as a revision aid to help with your exams.

Introduction

LEARNING OUTCOMES

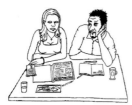

After studying this chapter you should be able to:

1 Describe the anatomical position

2 Describe the terms such as medial, lateral, proximal, distal and so on, included in this chapter

3 Be able to describe the planes of the body

4 Be able to describe the movements listed in this chapter, e.g. flexion, abduction, etc.

5 Be able to classify the types of synovial joint

6 Be able to classify types of bones

7 Know the functions of the skeleton

8 Be able to describe the features of bones listed

9 Be able to classify morphology of muscle

10 Be able to describe the function and components of a synovial joint.

FINDING YOUR WAY IN ANATOMY

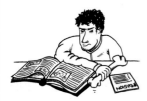

As with any long journey, you need to know your starting point. Anatomy has its own language and terminology, which is really not difficult once you understand the basics, that is what these next few pages are all about. Even before this, however, you need to understand an important concept.

Experiment . . .

Put your hand on the table palm downwards . . . . point to the top of your hand

Now place it palm up . . . . point to the top of your hand

Do you see the problem?

It is difficult to know which surface to call the top and which to call the bottom of the hand. A similar mix up in a patient lying on an operating table could have disastrous consequences. Therefore, in anatomy and medicine, all descriptions assume the ANATOMICAL POSITION; this is shown below.

THE ANATOMICAL POSITION

Person stands erect, facing forwards feet point forwards slightly apart, arms hanging down by the sides with palms facing forwards.

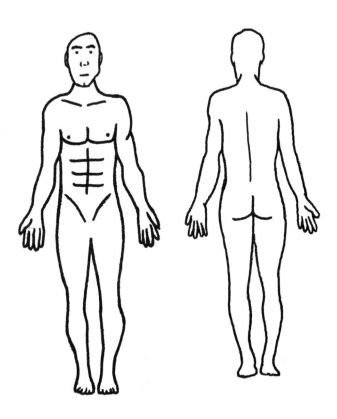

IS ALL OUR ANATOMY THE SAME?

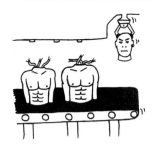

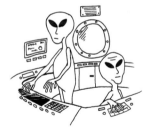

Thankfully we are all individuals with different appearances and characteristics. Being different gives each of us a unique identity of which we are proud. Yet at the same time, we all have the same design plans. You may find it strange to learn that there are anatomical differences from person to person. Some people have extra bones (not major ones). Some people have muscles that are absent in others, and a nerve that supplies a particular muscle in your arm may not be exactly the same as the same nerve in your friend's arm. All of these minor variations may be considered normal. However, we are basically put together in the same way, and the study of anatomy is possible, unless of course you end up working in outer space treating space aliens – I can't help you there!

Little green men may not have the same anatomy as you and me.

Introduction

DIRECTIONS IN ANATOMY

Now we have a map (anatomical position), we need some directions.

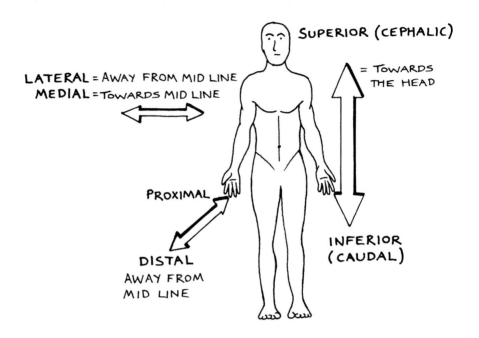

☞ Remember a piece of fluff in close proximity to your belly button (**umbilicus**).

☞ Remember painting your **fingernails a dist**urbing (distal) colour.

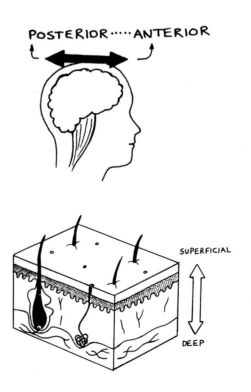

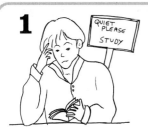

1 **From now on, whenever you see this symbol, it refers to projects that you need to study on your own.**

Find definitions for the following terms and put them into your own words.

| Inferior | Superior |

| Anterior | Posterior |

| Medial | Lateral |

| Prone | Supine |

| Deep | Superficial |

Note: combinations of words are sometimes used to describe positions, rather like compass points. So a cross between north and west is northwest, a cross between superior and lateral is superolateral. So, for example, your ear is superolateral to your mouth.

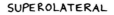
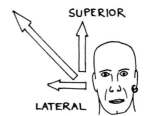

Important – no matter what position you put yourself in, all measurements in anatomy are taken from the anatomical position.

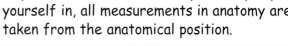

Introduction

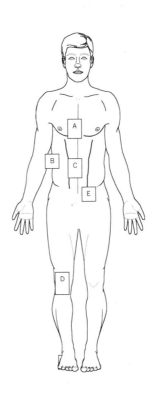

Place an ×:
Superior to letter A
Distal to letter B
Lateral to letter C
Proximal to letter D
Inferior to letter E
Inferomedial to
letter A.

THE PLANES OF THE BODY

If we take a human body we can
cut it in various directions.

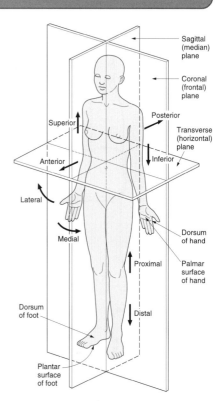

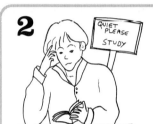

2 Using anatomical terminology, describe these three sections of the head.

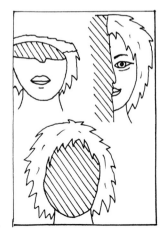

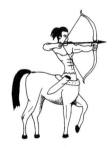

Remember Sagittarius the Archer firing an arrow directly at you, the arrow would pass through you in a sagittal plane.

Important point: in anatomy 'the leg' refers to the knee downwards, including the foot. The part between the hip and the knee is called the thigh.

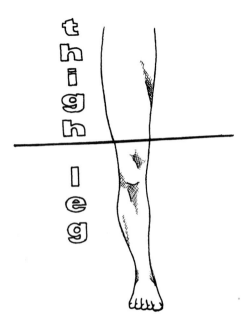

Introduction

This does not really matter when you are speaking to your patients but in examinations and assignments you should use the correct terminology.

On the subject of exams, never write *I think... You* can... *It's got...* or abbreviate, e.g. 'quads'. You should state 'quadriceps femoris'. Abbreviations tend to annoy examiners unless you first define them; for example, the anterior cruciate ligament (ACL). You can then use ACL without being penalised. Only use abbreviations or bullet points if you are running out of time.

MEET JENNY

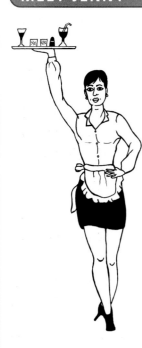

Jenny is a waitress. Try this fill in the blanks test to see if you understand anatomical terminology.

- Jenny wakes up in the morning. She is lying on her back, in a ①.................... position.
- She sits up and looks at her watch. She notices that her fingernails need cutting. Her fingernails are ②.................... to her wrists.
- She goes into the bathroom and cleans her teeth. She notices a pain in her shoulder, which is ③.................... to her elbow.
- She looks in the mirror and wishes she had not been partying last night, she has bags under or ④.................... to her eyes.
- She plucks her eyebrows which are ⑤.................... to her eyes.
- She goes to work and her first job is to lift a tray of drinks above her head. In this position her hand is ⑥.................... to her elbow and ⑦.................... to her shoulder.
- She then puts her arm down to her side. In this position her hand is ⑧................ to her elbow and ⑨................ to her shoulder.
- As she is serving, she bangs her thigh on the table. Later she notices a bruise on the outside of her thigh, or on the ⑩.................... aspect.

Answers

① supine. ② distal or inferior. ③ proximal or superior. ④ inferior. ⑤ superior. ⑥ inferior or distal. ⑦ inferior or distal. ⑧ same as ⑥. ⑨ same as ⑦. ⑩ lateral. ⑦ and ⑧ were trick questions, the position of her hand is irrelevant, her hand will always be distal to her shoulder no matter what she does with it!

10

MOVEMENTS IN ANATOMY

Movements in an antero-posterior direction (i.e. median or paramedian plane)

(DO NOT FORGET THAT ALL MOVEMENTS ARE IN RELATION TO THE ANATOMICAL POSITION.)

☞ **Flexion**   The bending of two body segments so that their two anterior or posterior surfaces are brought together.

☞ **Extension**   Movement in the opposite direction to flexion.

☞ **Plantarflexion**   For the ankle, this refers to pointing the foot downwards (when wearing stilettos your foot is plantarflexed). Pulling the foot towards the body is dorsiflexion.

Movements in a lateral direction (i.e. in a coronal plane)

☞ **Abduction**   Movement of a body segment away from the mid-line.

☞ **Adduction**   Movement opposite to abduction.

☞ **Lateral flexion**   The term used to describe sideways bending of the trunk to the left or the right.

☞ **Circumduction**   A combination of all movements, e.g. the shoulder circumducts when you swim the crawl (it moves in a cone). This is commonest at the hip and shoulder joints.

Rotation

Movement of a bone around a central axis without displacement of that axis is rotation, it may be inward (medial/internal) or outward (lateral/external).

☞ **Supination**   This describes the act of turning the palm towards the ceiling when standing (it is also occasionally used to describe movements in the foot).

☞ **Pronation**   The opposite of supination, where the palm is turned down towards the floor.

Special movements

Some movements do not fall into any of the above categories.

☞ **Elevation**   Raising a part, e.g. shrugging your shoulders is elevation of the shoulder girdle.

☞ **Depression**   The opposite to elevation.

☞ **Protraction**   Moving a part forwards, e.g. rounding your shoulders.

☞ **Retraction**   The opposite to protraction.

☞ **Inversion**   Turning the sole of your foot inwards as if looking at your sole is inversion.

☞ **Eversion**   The opposite to inversion.

11

THE MAIN TYPES OF SYNOVIAL JOINT

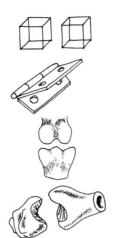

PLANAR
E.G. INTERTARSAL JOINTS OF THE FOOT.
YOUR NOTES

HINGE JOINT
YOUR NOTES

BICONDYLAR / BICONDYLOID
E.G. THE KNEE JOINT.
YOUR NOTES

SADDLE JOINT E.G. CARPOMETACARPAL JOINT AT THE BASE OF THE THUMB.
YOUR NOTES

ELLIPSOID
YOUR NOTES

SPHEROID (BALL-AND-SOCKET)
E.G. THE HIP JOINT.
YOUR NOTES

CLASSIFICATION OF BONES

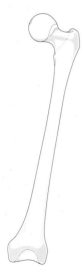

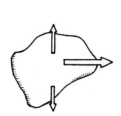

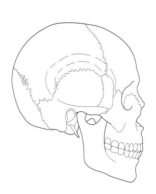

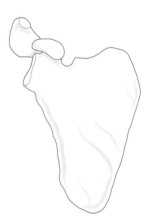

Long bones, e.g. femur or humerus (longer than they are wide).

Short bones, e.g. cuboid in the foot (do not have a long axis).

Flat bones, e.g. bones of the skull.

Irregular bones, e.g. scapula (shoulder blade) and pelvis (don't fit any category).

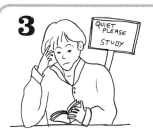

3

☞ Look in a butcher's shop window – what colour is a fresh bone?
☞ When you start looking at skeletons in the classroom, you will notice that they are chalky and white. Why?
☞ Why is a broken bone painful?

Answers

☞ Living bone is pink.
☞ Classroom skeletons have lost their organic parts; all that remains are hard mineral salts.
☞ Bone is alive, highly vascular and surrounded by a sensitive membrane – the periosteum.

THE TASKS OF THE SKELETON

Millions of years ago, humans opted for an endoskeleton (internal). This has good and bad points, but at least we don't have to shed our skeleton whenever we wish to grow, like insects do.

Our skeleton has these functions:

1 Support – the framework of the body, most muscles attach to bones

2 Movement – bones end in joints, so the shape of the bones often dictates how we can move

3 Protection – vital organs such as the brain are encased in bone, lungs are encased by ribs, and the uterus in the female is protected by the bowl of the pelvis

4 Mineral reservoirs of calcium, phosphorus, sodium, potassium and so on, are stored in bone. They can be moved around and mobilised when necessary, e.g. calcium is removed from the bones of the pregnant mother to give to the foetus. This is an important point since osteoporosis is an increasingly common condition. This is where the bone begins to lose mineral density either through lack of weight-bearing exercise (e.g. a patient on bed rest, or in a wheelchair) or through hormonal changes

5 Haemopoiesis (red marrow produces red blood cells).

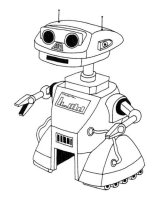

An external (exoskeleton) would look cool but you would need to shed it to grow – ask any insect what a pain that is!

Introduction

FEATURES OF BONES

Projections	For articulation with other bones
	    Head, condyle, facet
	For ligament/muscle attachment
	    Trochanter
	    Tuberosity
	    Epicondyle
	    Tubercle

Elongated projections	Process Spine Ramus
Ridges	Crest Line Ridge Spine

Depressions	Facet
	    Smooth, slight depression
	Fossa
	    Depression
	Fovea
	    Pit for ligament attachment
	Sulcus
	    Groove or channel

Holes	Foramen = hole Meatus = canal

4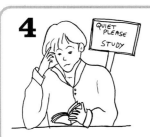

- Look through your Palastanga anatomy book and find one example of each of the terms on the previous page.
- All bones have these various lumps and bumps. How can an archaeologist tell by looking at a femur whether the person was a muscular individual?
- Why am I so keen for you to know where they are?

Answers

- Bones possess lumps and bumps in response to attachment of ligaments, muscles or tendons. Basically if a bone possesses a bump – something attaches to it!
- An archaeologist or forensic scientist can estimate how muscular an individual was by examining the size and development of bony prominences; bodybuilders for example will have larger bumps than inactive people such as lecturers!
- You need to know what is normal before you can hope to identify the abnormal.

COMPONENTS OF A MUSCLE

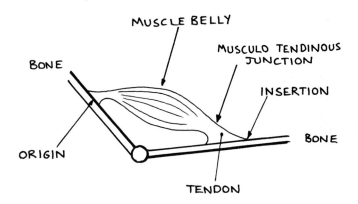

Connective tissue coverings (fascia)

Each skeletal muscle is composed of many separate fibres; these are bound together by sheets of connective tissue called fascia. The fascia that encases an entire muscle is called the epimysium. Fascia also penetrates muscle, separating muscle fibres into bundles called fasciculi.

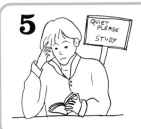

5 Make your own notes on fascia – its composition and properties.

Introduction

Muscles are anchored to the skeleton by extensions of the layers of fascia enveloping and within them. These extensions may attach directly to the periosteum (bone lining) or they may blend into a strong fibrous connection (tendons). Tendons may be quite short or may be up to 30 cm long; tendons that take the shape of broad sheets are called aponeuroses.

MORPHOLOGY (SHAPES) OF MUSCLES

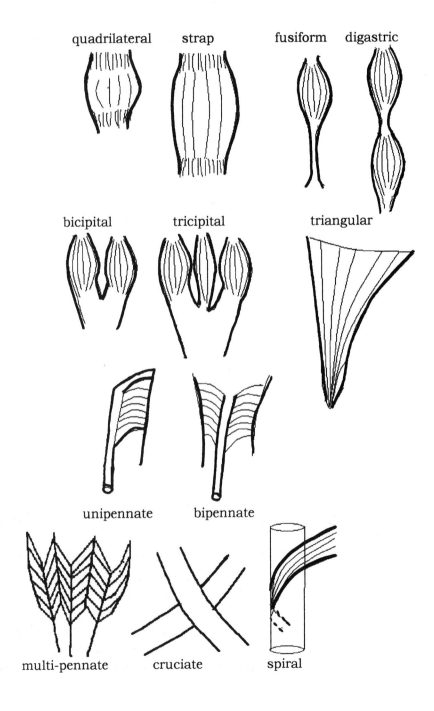

quadrilateral   strap   fusiform   digastric

bicipital   tricipital   triangular

unipennate   bipennate

multi-pennate   cruciate   spiral

6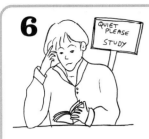

Think about it.

When a muscle contracts, it shortens in length and pulls its ends closer together. If the muscle is attached to either end of two bones, it pulls their ends closer together.

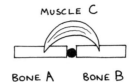

Below I want you to draw how bones A and B would look when muscle C contracts...

1 If bone A is immobile

2 If bone B is immobile

3 If both bones are immobile

Answers

☞ If bone A is immobile, bone B will move in an arc around the central joint.

☞ If bone B is immobile, bone A will move in an arc around the central joint.

☞ If both bones are immobile, then the net result will be compression at the joint. Muscles often work. simultaneously across joints to give them stability, e.g. biceps and triceps in the arm.

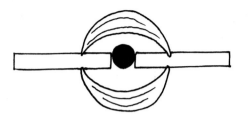

If both muscles above contract simultaneously, what will be the effect on the joint in the centre?

Answer   Joint stabilisation.

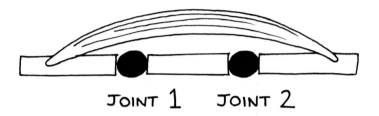

JOINT 1   JOINT 2

A. If this muscle contracts, what will it do to joints 1 and 2?

Draw the result below.

B. Draw the position into which you would put the bones if you wished to stretch or even snap (rupture) the muscle.

Answers

A.

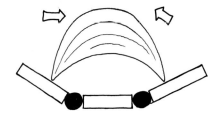

B.

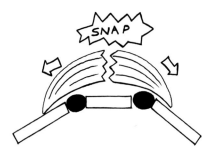

TYPES OF MOVEMENT

This can take a little effort to grasp so I would like you to meet Fred. Fred is a student. I will use a 1-hour period in his life to attempt to explain various types of joint movement.

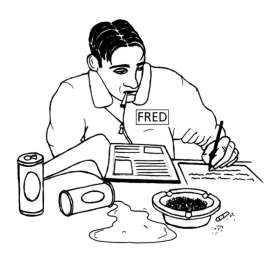

Fred was up studying until 2.00 a.m. (As all students do!)

He has an exam today.

He is so tired he fell asleep with his arm on his textbook last night.

His flatmate needs the book and so, without waking Fred, the flatmate lifts up Fred's arm and removes the book.... This is an example of a **passive movement** on Fred's part. It required no muscle action by Fred even though Fred's shoulder joint moved.

Fred begins to wake up but he is late for the exam, his friend helps to dress him and helps him to lift his arm into his pullover, Fred does some of the work and so does his friend…. This is an example of an **active assisted movement**. Fred's own muscles did some but not all of the work.

Fred is now in the bathroom and reaches up to grab the toothpaste …. This is an **active movement** – Fred's own muscles controlled the movement.

Fred now rushes down the hall and tries to open the door, it sticks and he has to push it quite hard…. This is a **resisted movement** – Fred's muscles had to work against an external force.

(Fred passed his exam.)

Please note that any similarity to any student living or dead is purely coincidental. No student would ever be so silly as to leave revision this late or oversleep for an exam … would you … hello …?

TYPES OF MUSCLE WORK

There now follows a practical demonstration involving something very dear to my heart – food.
   You will need

   1. A meat pie.

Let us look at a single muscle, in this case the biceps brachii.

At rest, the muscle is relaxed and generates no tension.

Lift the pie towards your mouth, the biceps contracts and flexes your elbow.

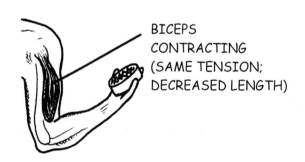

BICEPS
CONTRACTING
(SAME TENSION;
DECREASED LENGTH)

During this movement, the biceps shortens in length. This is called a *concentric* contraction. As you lower your arm back down to replace the pie (extend the elbow) it is still the same muscle doing the work but this time it is slowly paying out tension and thus lengthening. This is an *eccentric* contraction. Concentric and eccentric contractions are collectively termed isotonic contractions because there is a change in the length of the muscle.

Now, let's assume that the pie has been glued to the table – a distressing concept I know. You try to pick it up and you can feel the tension and see the contraction in the biceps, but the pie does not move, and the elbow remains motionless: this is called an *isometric* contraction. The muscle has contracted but has not changed in length.

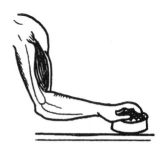

So, to summarise the types of muscle contraction

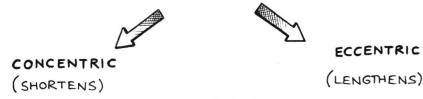

ISOTONIC
(CHANGE IN MUSCLE LENGTH)

CONCENTRIC
(SHORTENS)

ECCENTRIC
(LENGTHENS)

ISOMETRIC
(NO CHANGE IN MUSCLE LENGTH)
TENSION IS STILL GENERATED

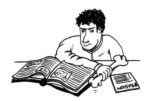

How can I remember what an eccentric contraction looks like?

Imagine one of your *eccentric* lecturers who is handing an assignment back to you, he slowly *lowers* the assignment on to the table suggesting that maybe you should be *paying* for extra tuition, whilst trying to control his rage – this is an *eccentric* contraction of the biceps as it slowly controls the movement and *pays* out its length.

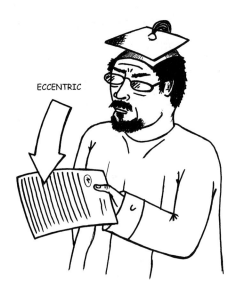

ECCENTRIC

BURSA (PLURAL BURSAE)

Rub hands together – what happens? – they get hot, keep doing this all day and you would quickly wear away your skin.

Now, put a bottle of ketchup or a can of cola between your hands and rub them as you did before, what happens?

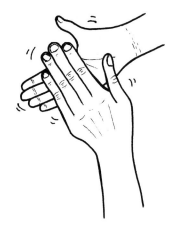

1 The can or bottle rolls with your skin
2 Your hands do not get hot
3 You could keep going all day without wearing away your skin.

This is the best way I can think of to describe how a bursa works. A bursa is an expansion of synovial membrane that is found at sites of potential friction, e.g. between your Achilles tendon and your calcaneus (heel bone). Bursae are lubricated on their inner walls by synovial fluid.

By rolling between the two structures, friction is kept to a minimum and damage is prevented – think about how many thousands of times per day your tissues might rub against one another.

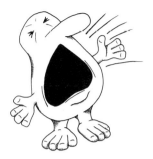

Meet Billy Bursa. As you can see, he is inflamed. This is known as bursitis.

What would you have to do to him to make him irritable?

1 Stretch him	**4** Infect him
2 Overuse him	**5** All of the above
3 Squash him	**6** None of the above.

Answer – all of the above could give Billy bursitis.

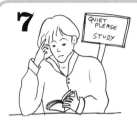

7 What are the symptoms of bursitis?

COMPONENTS OF A TYPICAL SYNOVIAL JOINT

You *must* know the function of each of these structures in a normal joint before you can understand how they are affected by various conditions and diseases.

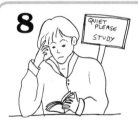

8 **What are the functions of these structures? The more you do now, the less you have to do before your exams!**

Muscle

Cartilage

Synovium

Ligament

Nerve

Tendon

Joint capsule

Meniscus

Bursa

Judgement time

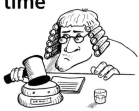

How have you done?

❑ It is now time for you to assess whether or not you have successfully achieved the learning outcomes that I set out at the start of this chapter.

❑ You need to be able to tick each box below.

❑ If you cannot, return to the study of the relevant section of the chapter.

❑ Can you describe the anatomical position?

❑ Can you describe the terms such as medial, lateral, proximal, distal and so on included in this chapter?

❑ Are you able to describe the planes of the body?

❑ Are you able to describe the movements listed in this chapter, e.g. flexion, abduction and so on?

❑ Are you able to classify the types of synovial joint found in the body?

❑ Are you able to classify types of bones?

❑ Do you know the functions of the human skeleton?

❑ Are you able to describe the features of bones listed?

❑ Are you able to classify morphology of muscle?

❑ Are you able to describe the function and components of a typical synovial joint?

❑ Can you recall the features of the bones listed?

Anatomy is a practical subject. You need to practise palpation (to examine medically by touch) on each other; you will be expected to undress down to bra and substantial underwear for the practical sessions.

You will probably get used to this very quickly and it is not as bad as it sounds. For some students, however, the thought of this a problem.

If you do not expose the model's body part in your practical examinations you may fail.

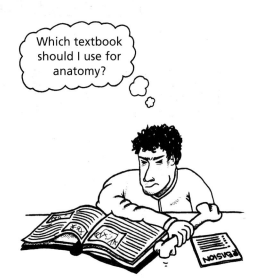

You need to buy this book

Palastanga, N., Field, D., Soames, R.
Anatomy and Human Movement. Structure and Function.
Butterworth-Heinemann. ISBN 0 7506 5241 1
(about £45).

Highly recommended
Field, D. *Anatomy Palpation and Surface Markings.*
Butterworth-Heinemann. ISBN 0 7506 4618 7
(about £25).

Highly recommended
Video Atlas of Human Anatomy, by Robert Acland. Lippincott
Williams & Wilkins. ISBN 0 683 18182 3 (×1 upper and ×1 lower
limb versions).

They are quite cheap – about £20 each. They do not give origins
and insertions of muscles, but are excellent if you learn well
using pictures and demonstrations. I would strongly recommend
these.

Other books/CD-ROMs
Interactive skeleton (Student version, CD-ROM Approx £30.
ISBN 1-902470-00-1). Excellent bone graphics, muscle attach-
ments and questions. www.Primalpictures.com.

The Anatomy Colouring Book, by Wynn Kapit & Lawrence M.
Elson. ISBN 0 06 455016 8.

BONES OF THE LOWER LIMB

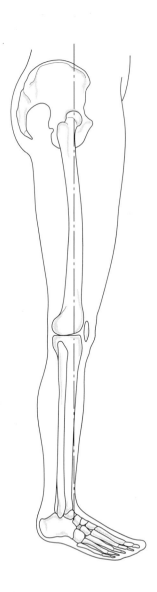

Bones of the lower limb

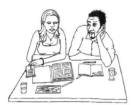

LEARNING OUTCOMES

In this chapter and the relevant theory/practical sessions you should be able to:

1 Describe in detail the structure and function of all of the bones of the lower limb.
2 Be able to palpate these bony points (on two models of different gender).

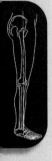

- ❏ ASIS
- ❏ PSIS
- ❏ iliac crest
- ❏ pubic tubercle
- ❏ ischial tuberosity
- ❏ greater trochanter
- ❏ adductor tubercle
- ❏ medial femoral condyle (plus epicondyle)
- ❏ lateral femoral condyle (plus epicondyle)
- ❏ medial tibial condyle
- ❏ lateral tibial condyle

- ❏ tibial tuberosity
- ❏ patella
- ❏ head of the fibula
- ❏ medial malleolus
- ❏ lateral malleolus
- ❏ tuberosity of navicular
- ❏ cuboid
- ❏ calcaneal tuberosity
- ❏ tubercle at base of 5th metatarsal
- ❏ metatarsals 1–5
- ❏ phalanges 1–5.

THE PELVIS

Anterior view

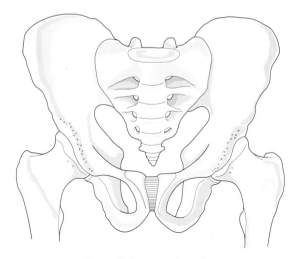

The pelvis anterior view

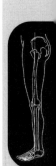

Three separate bones form the pelvis:

- the ilium
- the ischium
- the pubis.

The ilium is the broad, wing-like bone which features the wide, slightly concave surfaces of the back and sides of the pelvic girdle. The ischium forms the smaller, lower portion which bears the weight of the body while sitting. The pubis creates an archway in the front of the basin which allows the urethra, blood vessels and nerves to pass through the pelvic girdle to the external genitalia and lower body. The pelvis articulates with the sacrum in the back (and thereby connects to the rest of the vertebral column) and to the legs through the ball-and-socket joint formed by the acetabulum of the pelvis and the head of the femur.

THE PELVIS – PRACTICAL

1 Sit on your hands (rock from side to side). The bones you can feel are part of the ischium called the ischial tuberosity. You have two of these. The hamstring muscles attach here.

2 Put your hands on your hips. You are now resting your hands on top of part of your ilium called the iliac crest. You have two of these. These are large wing-like bones made up of cancellous or spongy bone; these are sometimes used by surgeons to harvest bone grafts for use in other parts of the body. Anteriorly the crests end at the anterior superior iliac spines (ASIS) and posteriorly at the posterior superior iliac spines (not surprisingly known as the PSIS!).

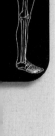

The innominate bone (left side)

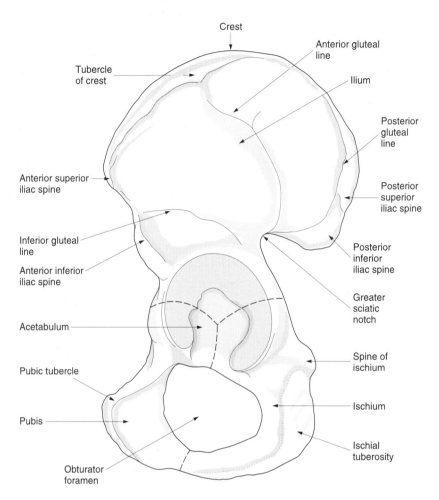

Crest

Anterior gluteal line

Tubercle of crest

Ilium

Posterior gluteal line

Anterior superior iliac spine

Posterior superior iliac spine

Inferior gluteal line

Anterior inferior iliac spine

Posterior inferior iliac spine

Acetabulum

Greater sciatic notch

Pubic tubercle

Spine of ischium

Pubis

Ischium

Obturator foramen

Ischial tuberosity

PROFESSOR'S TIP

Think of the ilium as a box with a spine at each corner.

PROFESSOR'S TIP

In your practical exams, if you are asked to locate a bony point, undress the model so that you can see and palpate the skin over the area. If you do not adequately expose the part, you will fail.

About the pelvis

The pelvis is an irregular bone. It is shaped differently in men and women, and is wider in women (sorry!). Because of this the elbow of a woman has what is known as a carrying angle, i.e. the elbow deviates away from the body to accommodate the wider pelvis.

The pelvis is joined together at the anterior (front) by the pubic symphysis and posteriorly (at the back) by the sacroiliac joints. These joints do not move much, except during pregnancy. In pregnancy, a hormone called relaxin is secreted which makes ligaments more lax, allowing the baby to pass more easily through the pelvic girdle. (This may be one of the reasons why back pain is more

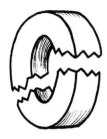

common during pregnancy. The pelvis may be regarded as a ring. If a ring breaks it breaks in two places (imagine snapping a polo mint) – the same is true of the pelvis.

The pelvis is the point where the spine joins onto the lower limbs. A large number of muscles and tendons attach to the pelvis and the pelvis is important for control of posture and balance. Trauma or osteoporosis may cause fractures (= breaks) around the pelvis. Another function of the pelvis is protection of the abdominal organs, and the socket of the hip joint (the acetabulum) is in the pelvis.

Think of the pelvis like a soup ladle containing spaghetti:

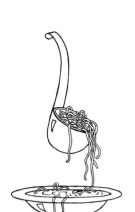

- the bowl = the pelvis
- the handle = the spine
- the spaghetti = abdominal contents
- in the same way that the bowl protects the spaghetti, the pelvis protects the viscera
- severe pelvic fractures may therefore have associated damage to the viscera (internal organs).

Add these labels to this diagram of a pelvis.

- pubis
- ilium
- ischium
- pubic symphysis
- pubic tubercle
- superior pubic ramus
- inferior pubic ramus

- acetabulum
- anterior inferior iliac spine (AIIS)
- anterior superior iliac spine (ASIS)
- posterior inferior iliac spine (PIIS)
- posterior superior iliac spine (PSIS)
- iliac crest
- obturator foramen.

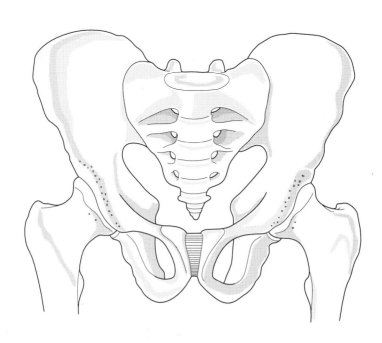

Bones of the lower limb

The sacrum

The sacrum is a wedge-shaped bone, which joins the pelvis via two joints on either side (the sacroiliac joints). These are synovial joints but unlike most others in that they consist of interlocking teeth with little or no movement occurring at the joint (although there is some disagreement about this fact). The sacrum is the portion of the vertebral column between the lumbar vertebrae and the structures of the coccyx. It is composed of five vertebrae which are fused together to form a single bone structure. Four pairs of holes (sacral foramina) pierce the sacrum, flanking the medial (centre) line, where the intermediate sacral crests are formed by the fused articular processes of the component vertebrae.

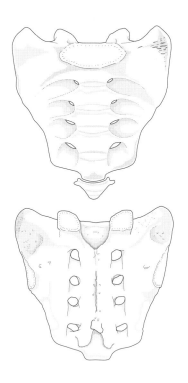

| COMPLETELY USELESS FACT NUMBER **256** | Apparently the sacrum is so called because when they used to burn witches at the stake it was always the last bone to burn, hence it was thought sacred. |
| | I guarantee that in times of stress, when your brain lets you down, you will remember odd facts like these! |

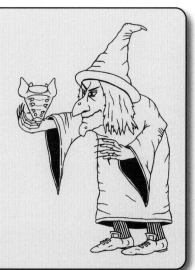

The coccyx

The coccyx is a vestigial tail. It is inferior to the sacrum. It is not really of importance except when playing Scrabble, or when it is fractured or bruised as after a fall onto the bottom. It is composed of three to five rudimentary vertebrae. Often, the first of these coccygeal vertebrae is separate, while the remainder are fused together. The articulation between the coccygeal vertebrae and the sacrum allows some flexibility in the coccyx.

In different colours on this lateral view of a pelvis and without looking at the rest of this workbook, draw the

- ilium
- ischium
- pubis.

(What does the term 'lateral' mean?)

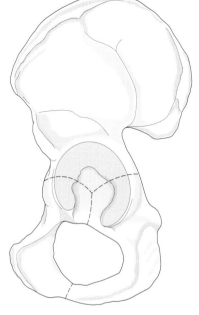

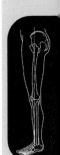

Now repeat the exercise on this anterior view.

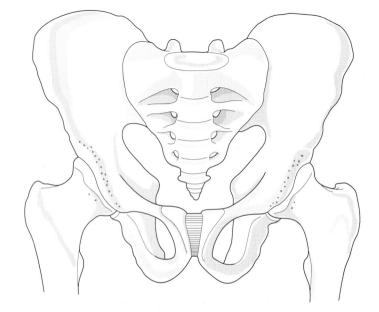

PROFESSOR'S TIP

Practise palpation on different bodies. We are all different and you need the experience.

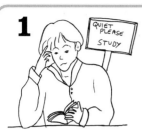

1 Give a detailed description of the bony structure of the pelvis.

Prompts

Where is it?
What type of bone is it?
What are its major features?
Which parts of the pelvis can be palpated?

Answer tips

☞ When answering this type of question, form a battle plan
☞ What are the key features of the bone and why is each feature there?
☞ What is the examiner looking for?
☞ This question is purely descriptive – so do not write essays on fractures of the pelvis, or the muscles or joints of the pelvis.
☞ Show your answer to a non-medical person – does it make sense to them?
☞ Do not use abbreviations and do not repeat yourself.
☞ Get out your highlighter pen and highlight the key words – in this case the key words are:

Detailed bony pelvis
☞ Keep re-reading the question.

THE FEMUR

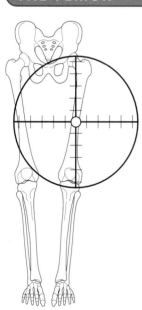

THE FEMUR (thighbone) is the longest bone in the body. Superiorly it forms the hip joint, inferiorly it forms the knee joint.

THE HEAD OF THE FEMUR is roughly spherical and is lined with articular cartilage; at the very top of this, a ligament (the ligamentum teres) attaches the head of the femur to the base of the socket of the hip joint (the acetabulum). The lining hyaline cartilage of the hip joint is frequently affected by degeneration (osteoarthritis). Hip replacement surgery is now very common and successful: it involves entirely replacing the head of the femur with a metal or ceramic prosthesis, and replacing the acetabulum with a tough plastic-like material. You will study joint replacement (arthroplasty) in greater detail in the future.

THE NECK OF THE FEMUR is what joins the head onto the shaft. It is important because it is one of the most common parts of the body to be affected by osteoporosis and therefore liable to fracture (break). This usually happens to the elderly who often have other conditions and may be generally frail – it is of vital importance that these fractures are fixed surgically and the patient is 'got back on their feet' as rapidly as possible.

THE SHAFT OF THE FEMUR is not straight. Hold a femur and look at it sideways on, note how it is bowed; this shape is stronger than a straight tube and aids shock absorption during activities such as running. Many muscles attach themselves around the shaft of the femur, most importantly the quadriceps or thigh muscles – these extend the knee. It takes considerable force to fracture a femur unless the bone is weakened by pathology such as a tumour or osteoporosis.

THE FEMORAL CONDYLES. A condyle is the term for a roughly rounded lump of bone, an epicondyle is the term for a lump on top of a condyle! The femur has two condyles, medial and lateral, you

Label this femur

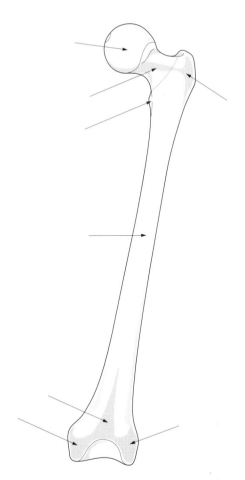

Left anterior view.

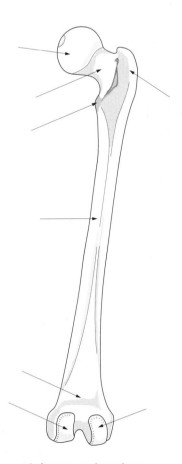

Right posterior view.

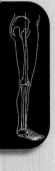

can feel them on your own knee. Just above the medial femoral condyle is a ridge of bone called the adductor tubercle to which attach the adductor or groin muscles. Put your hand between your knees and squeeze your thighs together: you can now see and feel your adductors working.

You should also be able to identify these parts of the femur: spiral line, linea aspera, quadrate tubercle, medial and lateral supra-condylar lines and the gluteal tuberosity.

PROFESSOR'S TIP

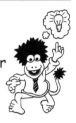

Fractures of the femoral neck are very common indeed and you will encounter them on clinical placement. Other common osteoporotic-related fractures include vertebral body and distal radial (Colles) fractures; these all consist predominantly of cancellous bone which is most affected by osteoporosis.

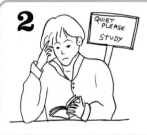

2

QUIET PLEASE STUDY

How does the structure of the femur relate to its function?

Answer tips

A slightly more advanced type of question than the pelvis one – a common exam format. Do not assume that because you have read the word femur that you are safe. This question asks for more than the structure. The examiner is asking you whether you can relate form to function. This is actually quite an easy task with anatomy since all form is there for a function. So what I would suggest is that you first make a bullet point list then go into more detail for the function of each.

Bullet point plan
- Spherical head → large range of movement (ROM)
- Articular cartilage → minimal friction
- Labrum → increased stability
- Offset femoral neck → larger ROM
- Large greater trochanter → powerful muscle attachment
- And so on.

Practical sessions are a vital part of your training, but take some getting used to. Please try not to feel too embarrassed in them – you are all in the same position and you will be surprised by how quickly you get used to them.

1 Sit in a circle in your tutorial groups. Pass round a pelvis and a femur. Each person says one thing – anything – about the bone

   e.g. 'it is long'
        'it is white'
        'it is irregular'.

Anything goes. There is no such thing as a silly answer. It is *very* important that you do not feel intimidated when speaking to the rest of your group. This gets much easier with practice. Work in twos and describe the pelvis and femur to each other. Now let your partner ask you questions about the bones and how they articulate in a living body.

2 Put your hands on your own hips. What can you feel? (bony points/soft tissues).

3 Spend a few minutes comparing what you can feel compared to a classroom skeleton. Now repeat this on your colleagues.

4 Sit on your hands. What are the hard bumps that you can feel?

5 Now repeat this on your colleagues.

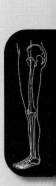

THE PATELLA (KNEECAP)

The patella is a small bone of the knee joint which resembles an inverted teardrop. It is a sesamoid bone, connected to the joint by the medial and patellar retinaculum ligaments and to the tuberosity of the tibia by the patellar ligament (poorly named as it is actually a tendon, not a ligament).

The patella is not there to act as a shock absorber. Its function is to act as a pulley, changing the angle of pull of the patellar tendon. Without a patella, the patellar tendon would approach the tibia virtually parallel to it, this would result in an inefficient system for extending the knee. The patella is the largest sesamoid bone in the body (a bone embedded within a tendon). The posterior surface of the patella has various facets which articulate with the femoral condyles throughout different parts of knee flexion/extension.

Bones of the lower limb

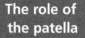

The role of the patella

A   Without a patella, the tibia would just 'crash head on' into the femur when the quadriceps contracted.

B   The patella alters the angle of attack of the patellar tendon, making knee extension more efficient.

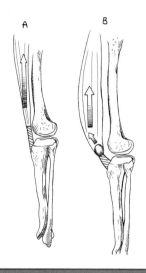

THE TIBIA AND FIBULA

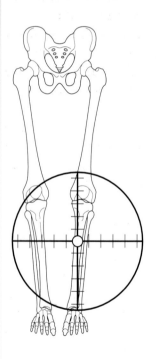

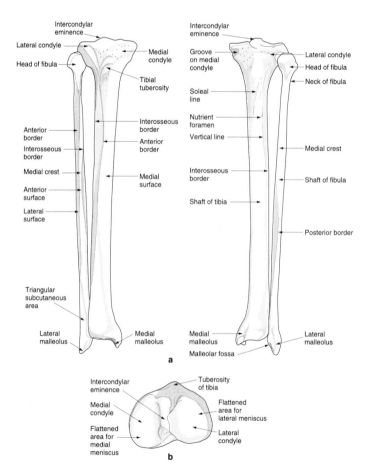

a) Right tibia and fibula, anterior view and posterior view.
b) Right tibia, superior view.

You should also be able to identify the following on a tibia: inter-condylar spines, lateral and medial condyles, Interosseous border, soleal line, vertical line, groove for flexor hallucis longus and the fibular notch.

Superiorly the tibia forms the inferior aspect of the knee joint, and inferiorly it makes up part of the ankle (talocrural) joint. Superiorly, it fans out into a broad platform known as the tibial plateau. On top of this is a lining of articular cartilage and two fibrocartilagenous discs called menisci (singular meniscus).

Working down the anterior border of the tibia one sees a large bump on the anterior aspect; this is called the tibial tubercle or tuberosity. This is where the patellar tendon attaches (the ligamentum patellae). You will find these types of lumps and bumps wherever powerful muscles or tough ligaments attach. These bumps are larger in men owing to their larger musculature and are even larger in bodybuilders. If you have ever had Osgood–Schlatter's disease, this is inflammation of this part of the body – common in adolescent boys. You can clearly feel your own tibial tubercle about 6 or 7cm below the kneecap.

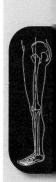

The anteromedial border is directly under the skin, which is why banging your shin hurts so much! The periosteum or membrane surrounding the bone is very sensitive to pain and has a good blood and nerve supply. (Never forget that bone is alive; a living bone is pink and vascular, not like the skeletons in the classroom which are white and chalky – have a look in a butcher's shop at fresh bones if you don't believe me.)

Inferiorly the tibia ends on the medial side in a rounded bone called the malleolus (plural malleoli); you can also feel this. The malleolus has a partner on the lateral aspect and together these grasp the talus, forming the ankle joint. The tibia is often fractured during sport or other accidents. Often the tibia fails to heal well because it has a poor blood supply, especially the distal portion – why do you think that is the case? The fibula is smaller and thinner than the tibia; it joins the tibia just below the tibial plateau and is sited lateral to the tibia and its main function is to act as a site of muscle attachment. It also makes up part of the ankle joint. Like the tibia it ends in a malleolus (lateral). The head of the fibula can be felt on the lateral aspect of the leg at approximately the same level as the tibial tubercle. It is possible to move the head of the fibula with your fingers but not a lot! The tibia and fibula are joined together by an interosseous membrane. The fibula is so named because it serves as a brace for the lower leg (fibula means 'brace').

Bones of the lower limb

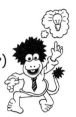
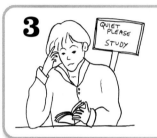

3

Describe the tibia and fibula on a page of A4.

THE FOOT

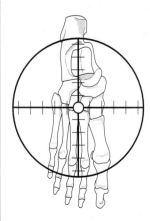

Each foot is made up of 26 bones; seven of these bones form the tarsus. These tarsal bones include the navicular, the three cuneiforms, the cuboid, the talus, and the calcaneus (which also forms the heel). These tarsal bones are arranged generally in two rows, the proximal (nearer the body) and distal (nearer the toes). The distal tarsals articulate with the five metatarsals. The long metatarsals form the broad, long structure of the foot. These, in turn, articulate with the proximal phalanges (toe bones). The proximal phalanges join with the middle phalanges, which articulate with the distal phalanges. The large toe is the exception, as it lacks a middle phalanx.

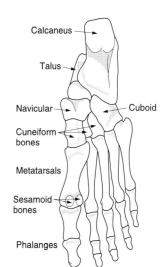

Right foot

Superior aspect

Inferior aspect

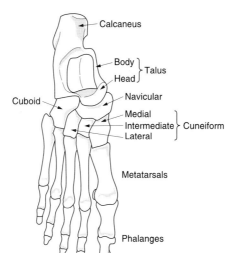

Calcaneus

Body
Head } Talus

Cuboid

Navicular

Medial
Intermediate } Cuneiform
Lateral

Metatarsals

Phalanges

Calcaneus

Talus

Navicular

Cuboid

Cuneiform
bones

Metatarsals

Sesamoid
bones

Phalanges

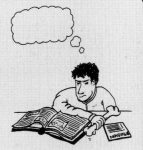

USELESS FACT NUMBER 462

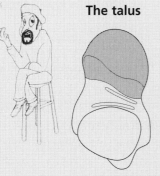

The talus

The talus from below – find the three facets for articulation with the upper surface of the calcaneus, and the articulation with the navicular bone.

The talus is the only bone in the body which has no muscle attachments.
Try that one at the next party you go to – it will really get things going!

The calcaneus

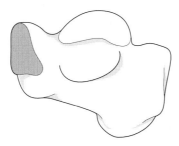

The right calcaneus.

Put an arrow on the diagram indicating the direction of:
1 The toes
2 The ankle joint
3 Find the sustentaculum tali and label it
4 Find the calcaneal tuberosity.

This shows the calcaneus from below (inferior view) – label it.

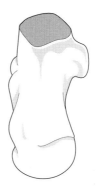

4 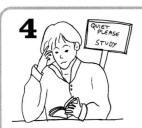 On the next pages there are diagrams of each of the tarsal bones, make your own notes on them in the spaces provided.

The calcaneus

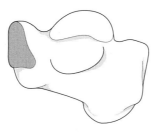

Often fractured by falls from a ladder onto the heels by:

☞ burglars
☞ window cleaners
☞ peeping toms!

Largest foot bone.

Transmits weight through the heel. Articulates with talus above and cuboid in front.
Your notes

USELESS FACT NUMBER 453

A patient (ex-sailor) once told me that during World War 2 the calcaneus was commonly fractured when a battleship was torpedoed – the shock being transmitted through the deck of the ship upwards through the heels – now you know.

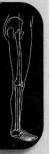

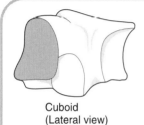

Cuboid
(Lateral view)

Your notes

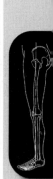

The cuboid

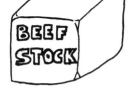

The cuboid looks a little like an Oxo cube
OK may be not
On the lateral side, it has a groove underneath to house the tendon of peroneus longus.

Your notes

The navicular

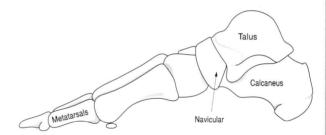

Talus

Calcaneus

Metatarsals

Navicular

The tuberosity of navicular can be palpated on the medial side of the foot.

Your notes

The cuneiforms

Your notes

CUNEIFORM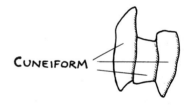

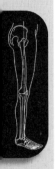

Bones of the lower limb

The metatarsals   Your notes

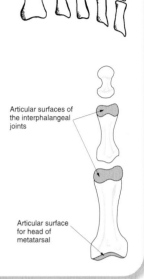

Articular surfaces of
the interphalangeal
joints

Articular surface
for head of
metatarsal

The phalanges   Your notes

5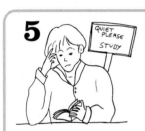

On a page, summarise the number, position and functions of
the arches of the foot.

THE ARCHES OF THE FOOT

**How muscles
assist in arch
support**

There are three main arches, a medial and lateral longitudinal and
a transverse arch. They are made up from the shape of the bones
and soft tissues, and muscles assist in maintaining their shape.

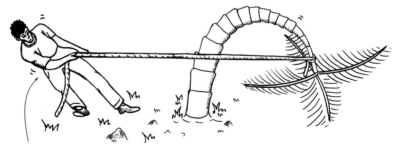

Muscles such as flexor hallucis longus.

Last time that you made an igloo you will remember that the way to get the blocks to rest securely on each other is to make them wedge shaped with the narrow part lowermost

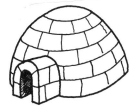
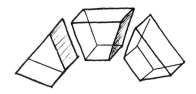

This is how the bones of the foot are shaped thus helping maintain an arch shape

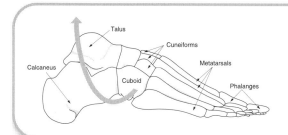
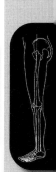

Talus

Cuneiforms

Calcaneus

Metatarsals

Cuboid

Phalanges

As well as the shape of the bones, ligaments and muscles act to support the shape e.g. peroneus longus

PROFESSOR'S TIP

Believe it or not, by the time you have been studying for a couple of months, you will know more anatomy than most patients *ever* will. Don't forget that in terms of knowledge, most patients never get past day 1 and are just as nervous and unsure as you were. So try to explain things to them in simple terms that *they* can understand – after all – that is how you remember things best isn't it?

6 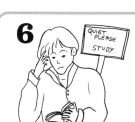 **On this leg, plot the bony points that you have learned to palpate so far.**

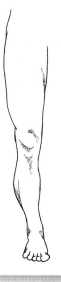

Here is a guide.

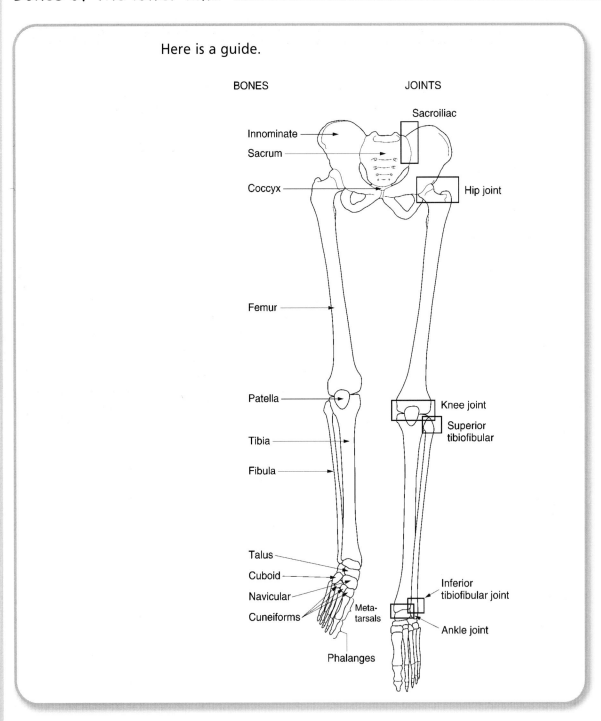

BONES   JOINTS

Sacroiliac

Innominate

Sacrum

Coccyx   Hip joint

Femur

Patella   Knee joint

                                          Superior
                                          tibiofibular

Tibia

Fibula

Talus
Cuboid   Inferior
Navicular   tibiofibular joint
Cuneiforms   Meta-
                tarsals   Ankle joint

        Phalanges

HOW MUCH DETAIL DO YOU KNOW?

Theory

You need to be able to describe and identify all the features of bones included in this chapter (including self-directed work).

Practical – bony points and landmarks

You must be able to find these points on models of various shapes and sizes!

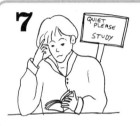

On three different models, find each of the bony points and get a colleague to check that you are correct.

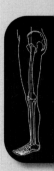

Bony point	Model 1	Model 2	Model 3
ASIS			
PSIS			
Iliac crest			
Pubic tubercle			
Ischial tuberosity			
Greater trochanter			
Adductor tubercle			
Medial femoral condyle (plus epicondyle)			
Lateral femoral condyle (plus epicondyle)			
Medial tibial condyle			
Lateral tibial condyle			
Tibial tuberosity			
Patella			
Head of the fibula			
Medial malleolus			
Lateral malleolus			
Tuberosity of navicular			
Cuboid			
Calcaneal tuberosity			
Tubercle at base of 5th metatarsal			
Metatarsals 1–5			
Phalanges 1–5			

Judgement time

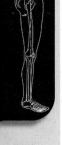

It is now time to see whether you have successfully achieved the learning outcomes listed at the start of this chapter. You need to be able to tick each box below before progressing further. If you cannot, return to the relevant section of this chapter before you move on to the next chapter.

❑ Can you describe in detail the structure and function of all of the bones of the lower limb?

❑ Can you accurately palpate these bony points?

❑ ASIS
❑ PSIS
❑ iliac crest
❑ pubic tubercle
❑ ischial tuberosity
❑ greater trochanter
❑ adductor tubercle
❑ medial femoral condyle (plus epicondyle)
❑ lateral femoral condyle (plus epicondyle)
❑ medial tibial condyle
❑ lateral tibial condyle

❑ tibial tuberosity
❑ patella
❑ head of the fibula
❑ medial malleolus
❑ lateral malleolus
❑ tuberosity of navicular
❑ cuboid
❑ calcaneal tuberosity
❑ tubercle at base of 5th metatarsal
❑ metatarsals 1–5
❑ phalanges 1–5.

❑ Can you identify the bony attachments/origin and insertion of the muscles and ligaments listed in the 'Joints of the lower limb' and 'Muscles of the lower limb' chapters?

JOINTS OF THE LOWER LIMB

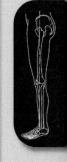

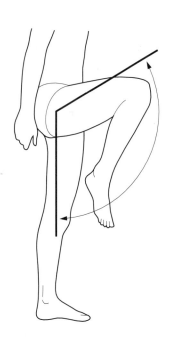

Joints of the lower limb

LEARNING OUTCOMES

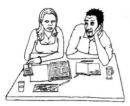

Read this before commencing your study of the joints of the lower limb

Upon completion of this workbook, the relevant lectures & practical sessions, you should be able to:

1 Describe the structure of all joints of the lower limb including articular surfaces, movements possible, ligaments, capsule and other important features particular to that joint.
2 Describe the function of all joints of the lower limb.
3 Be able to relate 1 (above) to 2 (above).
4 Have a working knowledge of limiting factors to movements of the joints of the lower limb.

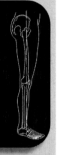

THE HIP JOINT

The hip is a remarkable joint which possesses stability but retains mobility. It has to withstand incredible pressures during life – 18 Mpa (2610 PSI) going up stairs for example. To put this in context, your car tyres typically use pressures of 200 kPa (29 PSI).

If you wish to learn in greater detail about this joint try this book: *The Hip Handbook* by Timothy L. Fagerson, Butterworth-Heinemann, ISBN 0 7506 9689 3.

Label this diagram of a hip joint.

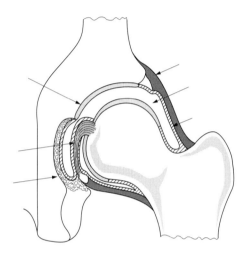

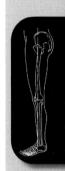

Left hip joint – coronal section.

The ligaments of the hip

Label the Ligaments.

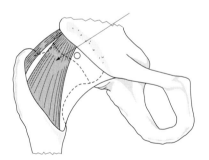

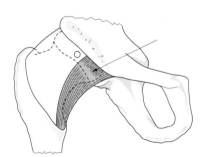

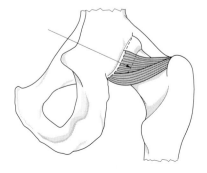

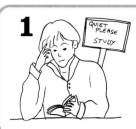

1 On the above, label the following ligaments and add notes on their attachments below.

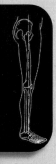

Iliofemoral ligament	(the strongest ligament in the body). It is not sufficient to say that it goes from the ilium to the femur. The only time this is OK is when you are having a 'no brainer' in your practical exam and you cannot think of anything else to say – in cases like this state the obvious.

Attachments

Function

Pubofemoral ligament

Attachments

Function

Ischiofemoral ligament

Attachments

Function

PROFESSOR ASKS

What would happen if a ligament became:

- ☞ Too lax?
- ☞ Too tight? (contracted)
- ☞ Snapped completely? (ruptured)
- ☞ Became inflamed or torn?

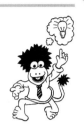

Answer tips

- ☞ Joint instability as is seen in degenerative joint disease where joint space is diminished resulting in the ligament effectively becoming too long to stabilise the joint.
- ☞ Loss of joint mobility.
- ☞ Major joint instability – oddly enough this is not always as painful as one might expect and may not be immediately diagnosed.
- ☞ Torn ligaments cause pain on stressing of the ligament, local tenderness on palpation and may cause joint effusions (swelling confined to a joint cavity).

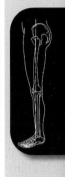

More on the hip joint

Rather like an egg in an eggcup, the hip joint is a ball-and-socket joint, it allows an infinite combination of movements yet keeps its stability.

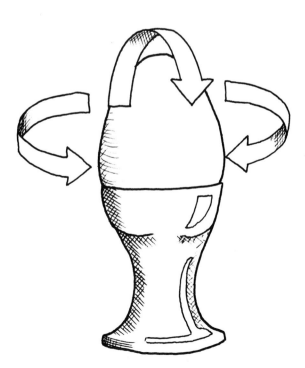

Add labels to these diagrams of the acetabulum and femur.

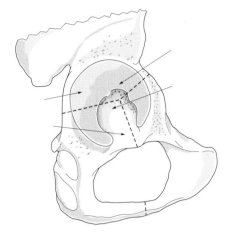

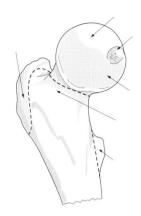

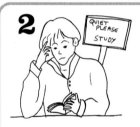

When you come to learn about the shoulder, the arrangement is a little similar but in the shoulder the eggcup does not make such a good job of containing the egg!

2 Make your own notes on:

THE ACETABULUM

THE HEAD OF THE FEMUR

THE ACETABULAR LABRUM

THE LIGAMENTUM TERES

THE ARTICULAR CARTILAGES of the femur/of the acetabulum

THE FOVEA

THE TROCHANTERIC BURSA

☞ Function

☞ Location

☞ Pathology.

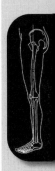

The surface marking of the hip joint

How to locate the joint on a model.

Find the mid point of inguinal ligament, go 1.5 cm inferior, this corresponds to the surface marking of the anterior of the hip joint.

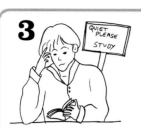

3 **Have a go!**

On these diagrams, draw the

☞ acetabular labrum

☞ inguinal ligament

☞ obturator membrane.

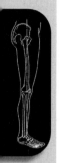

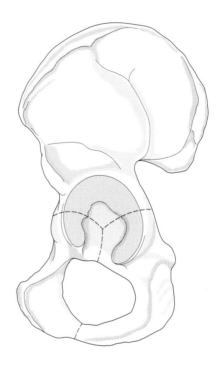

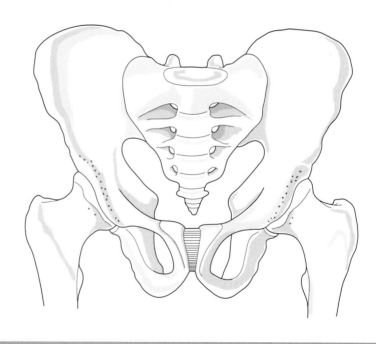

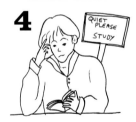

Movements at the hip joint

4

	Definition	Limiting factors to movement
Flexion		
Extension		
Abduction		
Adduction		
Internal (medial) rotation		
External (lateral) rotation		
Circumduction		

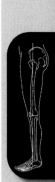

Note. Humans only have 10–15° of hip extension. Loss of hip extension is bad news, it affects the push-off phase of gait and means that a person cannot stand with a normal posture. It does not really make as much of a functional impact if one loses a few degrees of hip flexion.

Movements at the hip.

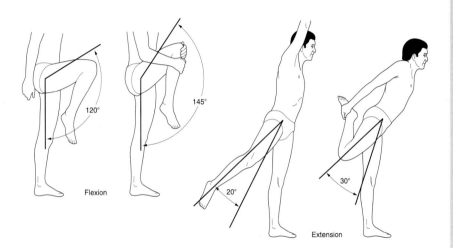

Joints of the lower limb

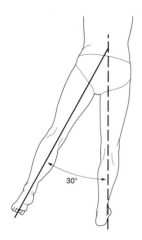

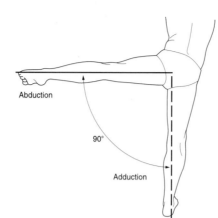

Abduction

90°

Adduction

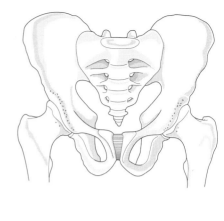

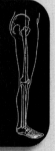

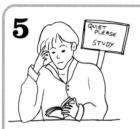

5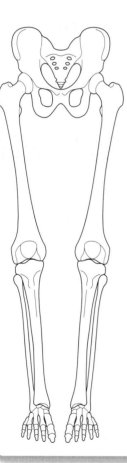

On your model and on the diagrams below locate the following.

Greater trochanter
Lesser trochanter (cannot really palpate this on a model and probably best not to try!)
Adductor tubercle.

❑ What and where is the ligamentum teres?
❑ What makes the socket of the hip joint deeper?
❑ Describe the blood supply to the femoral head.

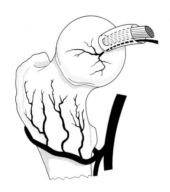

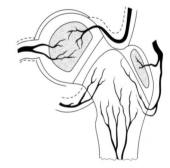

❑ Why does the femoral head sometimes die (avascular necrosis) following a badly displaced fracture or dislocation?
❑ State two similarities and two differences between the hip and the shoulder joints.

Similarities	Differences

Answers

The ligamentum teres is the internal ligament found within the hip joint. It might play a role in nutrition to the femoral head.

The blood supply to the femoral head is complex, most blood supply is from the periarticular anastomosis – this may be disrupted following fracture of the neck of the femur. Hence the risk of avascular necrosis (death of the femoral head from lack of blood).

Two similarities – both possess a labrum, both are spheroidal.

Two differences – one has internal ligament, one has two necks (humerus!).

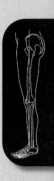

THE PUBIC SYMPHYSIS

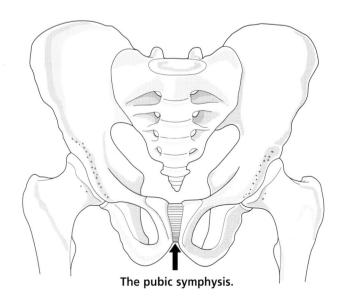

The pubic symphysis.

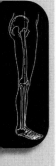

The two pubic bones meet in the median plane at the pubic symphysis. It is a cartilaginous joint with a disc in between the bones.

☞ Suprapubic ligament
☞ Arcuate pubic ligament
☞ Movements (not much except during childbirth).

Give three factors that make the hip joint very stable:

1.

2.

3.

Clues: depth of acetabulum, shape of bones, ligaments, muscles.

Give three factors that make the hip joint very mobile:

1.

2.

3.

Clues: type of joint, lining of bones, shape of femoral neck.

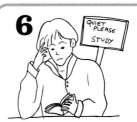

6

Let's talk

It is important that you practise describing things verbally, this gets much easier with practice, it will help in your practical exams and when you treat patients.
   Get a watch with a second hand or a stopwatch. Ask a fellow student to time you for five minutes. Talk for the *whole* five minutes about the hip joint. Ask your friend to score you on:

1 How interesting the talk was
2 How accurate the talk was
3 How much you hesitated
4 How confident they would feel if they were your patient?

Do this twice. First of all, talk to your friend as though they were a patient who has asked you what a human hip joint is like. Remember, patients usually do not know any anatomy. Then repeat the talk as though you were talking to a lecturer who knows everything (!) about the joint.

Repeat this for

☞ the knee
☞ ankle joint
☞ the small joints of the foot

when you have learned about them.

THE THOMAS TEST

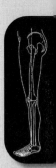

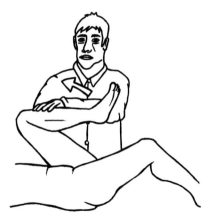

This is a demonstration of the Thomas test. The picture shows a positive result on the right leg. It is a test for a hip flexion deformity (contracture).

To test the right leg, perform passive hip and knee flexion on the opposite leg: a positive result occurs when the right hip flexes off the bed. Reason – at the extreme limit of hip flexion, the pelvis tilts posteriorly, i.e. the lumbar curve flattens.

If there is sufficient extensibility in the anterior structures of the hip, the leg will remain on the bed, if not, it will rise off the bed.

The other common test at the hip joint is the Trendelenberg test. Do you know what this test demonstrates?

Answer It is a test for weakness of the hip abductors – see 'gluteal gremlin' in the Muscles of the lower limb chapter.

Joints of the lower limb

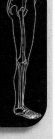

Bursae in the hip region

For each of the bursae below, find their location and function.

Trochanteric

Gluteal

Psoas

Typical anatomy questions

1 How does the structure of the hip joint relate to its function?
2 Give a detailed account of the muscles that abduct the hip and explain the signs and symptoms that result from weakness of these muscles.

Write a page on each of these.

☞ What are the key words to underline?
☞ What is the question asking?
☞ What will the examiner be looking for?
☞ What might be a common reason for some students to fail these type of questions?

THE KNEE JOINT

Get hold of a femur and a tibia and articulate them together as they would be in a living body (the most round part of the femoral condyles should be posterior, and the tibial tubercle should be anterior). Notice how they don't fit together as well as the femoral head did in the acetabulum. In fact if the knee only had bones to rely on for stability it would be very unstable! So what? Well, this should lead you to start thinking about what soft tissues might help the bones fit together a little better and give the knee joint some stability.

'Let's make a knee joint'

To help you understand some important concepts we are going to make a knee joint. You will need two eggs, a saucer, doughnuts and some water.

1 Lay the saucer on a table – this represents the superior aspect of the tibia.

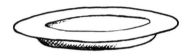

2 Put the eggs on top of the saucer – these represent the two femoral condyles.

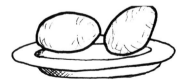

3 Notice how they roll around and end up laying on their side. This is because the radius of curvature of an egg is not uniform – look at a real femoral condyle – the same applies, the posterior portion of the condyle is a smaller diameter sphere than the inferior part. This means that when the knee is in a flexed position, it is inherently unstable, but when extended, the flat part of the condyle is in contact with the tibia. This is more stable and close packed (we will come back to this term in a minute).

Unstable   More stable

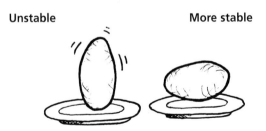

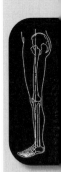

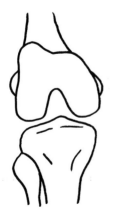

4 The problem is that the eggs still tend to roll around a little. So I now want you to put the two doughnuts on top of the saucer and rest an egg inside each. The doughnuts now represent menisci – they cradle the eggs, help them to become more stable and make the whole thing fit together better.

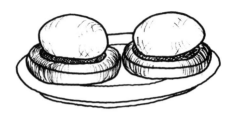

5 Now, if you wet the doughnuts to simulate synovial fluid and move the eggs around you will see that the doughnuts help more of the eggs' surface stay moist than the saucer alone could do. I know I'm rambling here but this is an important concept: articular cartilage relies on synovial fluid being swept over its surface to stay alive – this is called synovial sweep and it is another function of the menisci.

WHAT DOES 'CLOSE PACKED' MEAN?

Joints have some positions in which they are more stable than others. The position of maximum stability is when there is maximum contact between the articular surfaces and the surrounding ligaments are taut this is close packed. Think of it as a pop bottle with the top screwed on tightly. So for example the knee is close packed when extended, and the ankle is close packed when dorsiflexed.

The bare bones   Now, let us add the collateral ligaments and the menisci.

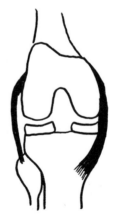

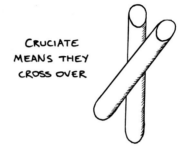

CRUCIATE MEANS THEY CROSS OVER

Now we add the cruciate ligaments.

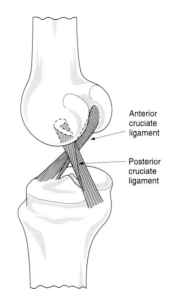

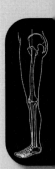

Anterior cruciate ligament

Posterior cruciate ligament

Location of anterior cruciate (ACL) and posterior cruciate ligaments (PCL).

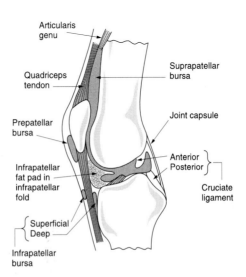

Articularis genu

Suprapatellar bursa

Quadriceps tendon

Joint capsule

Prepatellar bursa

Anterior
Posterior

Infrapatellar fat pad in infrapatellar fold

Cruciate ligament

Superficial
Deep

Infrapatellar bursa

The patella. A sesamoid bone. This is a bone that is embedded within a tendon.

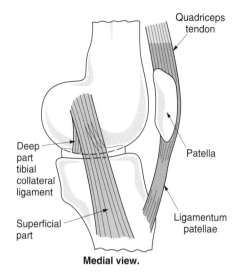

Deep part tibial collateral ligament

Superficial part

Quadriceps tendon

Patella

Ligamentum patellae

Medial view.

The medial tibial collateral ligament of the knee joint. Medial collateral ligament, a broad flat band, attached to medial meniscus so they may be injured together!

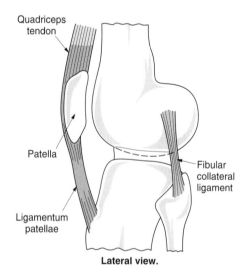

Quadriceps tendon

Patella

Ligamentum patellae

Fibular collateral ligament

Lateral view.

The lateral fibular collateral ligament of the knee joint.

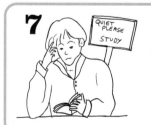

7 Describe the medial and lateral collateral ligaments of the knee to a friend who knows nothing about anatomy, explain to your friend what their role is, how they differ and their similarities.

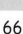

Medial collateral ligament	Lateral collateral ligament
Attachments/length	Attachments/length
Shape	Shape
Function	Function
Relationship to medial meniscus	Relationship to lateral meniscus

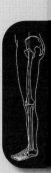

Answer tips

Classical examination question here.

The lateral collateral is cord-like and shorter than the medial collateral ligament and is not attached to the meniscus, unlike the medial collateral ligament.

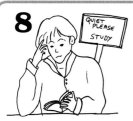

8 Complete this table

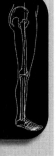

Medial meniscus	Lateral meniscus
Shape	Shape
Function	Function
Pathology	Pathology

Menisci in cross-section

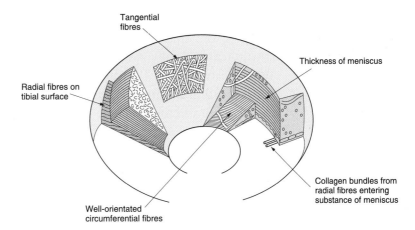

Diagram showing distribution of collagen fibres in the menisci of a knee.

Collagen is orientated in such a way as maximally to resist the forces brought to bear on the tissues. Most of the fibres are circumferentially arranged; a few are radially arranged, particularly on the tibial surface, these resist lateral spread of the meniscus. In the meniscus, tension is generated between the anterior and posterior attachments.

So what do the menisci do?

MENISCI ALLOW MAXIMUM CONTACT BETWEEN SURFACES AND SPREAD OF PRESSURE.

MENISCI REMOVED. DECREASED CONGRUENCY, DECREASED SYNOVIAL SWEEP AND LOSS OF SHOCK ABSORPTION.

The menisci are shaped like two croissants, sat on the tibia, but one is more circular than the other. The croissants are bound onto the tibia by coronary ligaments (like a crown). The croissants help the femur to fit onto the tibia better, and they also help synovial fluid wash over the femoral condyles thus feeding them; this is synovial sweep.

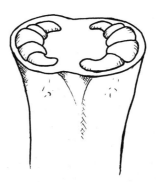

The croissant may tear along its length – longitudinal tear. If this happens, the loose flap lifts up like the handle on a bucket (bucket handle tear). It may also tear radially. Surgery to remove a meniscus is *menisectomy*. Peripheral tears of the meniscus may heal if sutured but sometimes it is just easier to remove the offending or frayed piece of croissant!

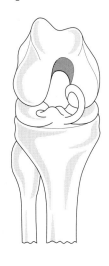 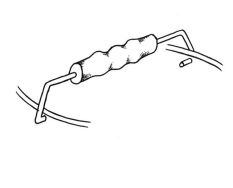

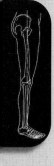

9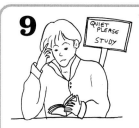

☞ From what you have learned so far about the location, structure and function of the menisci, think of the symptoms that you might expect in a patient who has a torn meniscus.

☞ Why do you think that the medial collateral ligament and medial meniscus are often injured simultaneously?

☞ What is the relationship of the popliteus muscle to one of the menisci?

☞ A patient who has sustained a ruptured anterior cruciate ligament runs a relatively high risk of sustaining a torn meniscus at a later stage – from what you have learned so far, hypothesise the reasons for this fact.

Answer tips

Torn meniscus = symptoms vary but possibly will complain of locking, giving way, recurrent effusions, loss of confidence, joint line tenderness, diffuse pain.

MCL and medial meniscus are connected therefore may be injured together.

Popliteus pulls the lateral meniscus out of the way during knee flexion – this might explain why it is injured less than its medial counterpart.

Ruptured ACL leads to abnormal knee biomechanics with increased shear forces on meniscus making it more liable to tear.

One of the functions of the menisci is to increase congruencey of the articular surfaces of the knee joint and to assist with synovial sweep (Aagaard & Verdonk (1999)).

This sounds impressive, doesn't it, but what does it mean?

1 Translate the statement into something which a patient with no anatomical knowledge could understand.
2 Then repeat as if you were answering a written question or an anatomy viva.

The functions of the menisci are load transmission and shock absorption, based on their collagen architecture, biochemical fluid composition, and their proteoglycan–collagen framework.

Stop press

Meniscal transplantation is now being recommended for certain meniscus-deficient patients (Rodeo 2001).

Varus and valgus at the knee

Which is which? This often causes confusion – but not any more.

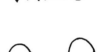

VARUS   VALGUS

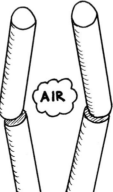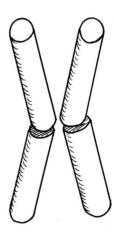

Just as there is air in between the varus knees, the word 'varus' has "air" in the middle – sort of! Oh well, suit yourselves – I tried.

The term *genu* is sometimes used for the knee so you might come across the terms *genuvarus* and *genuvalgus*.

The anterior cruciate ligament

Attachments are from the posterior aspect of the medial surface of the lateral femoral condyle, to the fossa just anterior and lateral to the tibial spines. Recent work shows it to be made of three separate bundles, which are orientated to resist stresses from multiple directions.

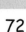

Its blood supply arises from the rich synovial fold which covers the ligament. One to 2% of the bulk of the ligament is neural tissue, containing Ruffini endings, Pacinian corpuscles, mechanoreceptors and free nerve endings. The proprioceptive role of the cruciates is vital.

Proprioception is the ability of the body to know its position in space.

Functions of the ACL

- It resists anterior tibial displacement on the femur
- It prevents hyperextension of the knee
- It controls and resists excessive rotation
- It fine-tunes the locking mechanism
- It acts as a secondary restraint against valgus and varus strain in all degrees of flexion
- Major role in proprioception (Fischer-Rasmussen & Jensen, 2000).

This is a representation of a PA draw test at the knee.

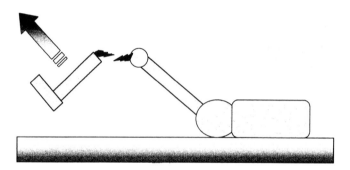

- Why is it PA?
- What does PA stand for?
- What would you suspect if the tibia moved too much in the direction of the arrow?

Answers

- Pulling back to front
- Posterior anterior
- Ruptured ACL.

The posterior cruciate ligament

Makris *et al.* (2000) have discovered four functionally distinct groups of fibre within this ligament:

- Anterior
- Central
- Posterior-longitudinal
- Posterior-oblique.

The overall effect of the arrangement of these fibre bundles is that no matter what the position of the knee, a portion of the ligament will always be under tension and therefore able to provide proprioceptive feedback and stability to the joint.

Attachments

From the depression in the intercondylar area of the tibia, it runs anteriorly, medially and proximally to the lateral surface of the medial femoral condyle.

Function (including) role in knee stability

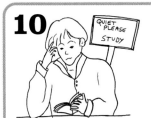

10 **What is proprioception?**

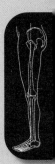

The coronary ligaments

Location

These attach the menisci to the edge of the tibial condyles.

Function

They help to hold the menisci in place.

The transverse ligament

Function

Joins the anterior portion of the menisci together.

Other ligaments in the knee

I will leave these up to you, e.g. arcuate popliteal ligament, etc. But:

☞ Make sure that you understand the functions and structure of the main four ligaments in the knee joint.

☞ Prepare a summary of the tests that may be used to test the integrity of the ACL/PCL medial and lateral collateral ligaments. You will return to this in more detail when studying soft tissue injuries.

Research the symptoms of patients who have ruptured (snapped) their anterior cruciate ligament – think about why they have each symptom. A pointer to get you started is that patients with a ruptured ACL lose proprioception in the affected knee joint (Fischer-Rasmussen & Jensen 2000).

11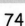

What is a bursa?

☞ Research three symptoms of bursitis (inflammation of a bursa).
☞ Work out why each symptom occurs.
☞ How would you describe a bursa to a patient?
☞ What is housemaid's knee?
☞ What is the infrapatellar fat pad?
☞ How far above the patella does the suprapatellar bursa extend?
☞ And why do you need to know this?

The patellar tap test

The knee has a large, expansive synovial membrane.

In injury or disease, one of the body's defence mechanisms is to produce more synovial fluid. If too much synovial fluid is produced it has nowhere to go except to float around inside the joint cavity. This is called an effusion. This is not the same as swelling which is not confined to a joint cavity.

If the effusion is large it can be seen (my knee swelled up like a football, Doctor!). If the effusion is less subtle, a test called the patellar tap test, can tell you if there is a mild effusion.

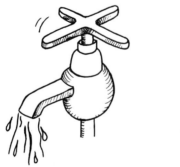
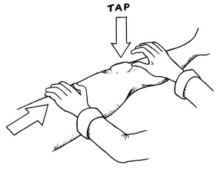

To perform the test, ask the patient to lie down, squeeze the fluid from the suprapatellar pouch (15 cm superior to the knee joint) by sliding your hand down towards the patella, and with your other hand bounce the patella on the femoral condyles. A tapping sensation or sound means there is an effusion.

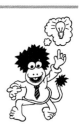

PROFESSOR ASKS

☛ What is oedema?
☛ What is swelling?
☛ What is effusion?

☛ If you sit on an aeroplane for 12 hours
☛ If you sprain your ankle
☛ If you undergo a total hip replacement
   – do you get oedema?
   – swelling?
   – effusion?

Movements at the knee joint

The knee is not simply a hinge (flexion/extension) it also has rotation; students often forget this. Don't forget that in anatomy you carry your syllabus around with you all the time.

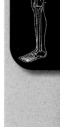

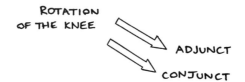

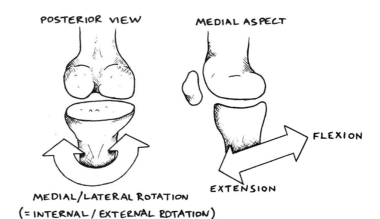

MEDIAL/LATERAL ROTATION
(= INTERNAL / EXTERNAL ROTATION)

Sit in a chair with your feet on the ground and your knees at a right angle. Rotate your feet inwards and outwards – this is adjunct rotation at the knee – a distinct movement that you do voluntarily.

Now extend your knee joint until your leg is straight – believe it or not you have just performed conjunct rotation – straightening the knee is not a straightforward hinge movement. In the final 30° of knee extension, the tibia rotates laterally on the femur. This allows close packing or full congruency of the joint. This is an involuntary movement that occurs without your control. Because of

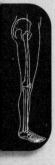

the shape of the femoral condyles and the tension in surrounding ligaments this would also happen in a cadaver's leg. The other way of putting this is that the femur rotates medially on the leg if the foot is fixed on the ground. Because of this, you need a special muscle (popliteus) at the posterior of the knee to unlock it from full extension.

Remember conjunct movement as your body is being <u>conned</u> into rotating beyond its voluntary control.

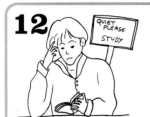

12 Describe the concepts of conjunct and adjunct rotation (as if you were doing a written exam, time yourself – 10 minutes).

Answer 10 minutes is not long. Get the important concepts across with an example of each. The thrust of the answer should be that conjunct is an automatic, involuntary movement whereas adjunct is under voluntary control.

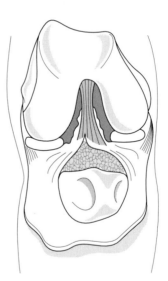

Inferior aspect of the femur, seen from below, and the posterior patellar surface.

☞ Occasionally, the patella does not track properly in the channel between the condyles of the femur, not surprisingly this is called a mal-tracking patella!

☞ What do you think the symptoms of this are?

☞ What is the Q angle? And how is it measured?

☞ Why do you need to know about it?

The knee – practical

Draw on your model:

☞ The medial and lateral femoral condyles (what is an epicondyle?)
☞ The medial collateral ligament
☞ The lateral collateral ligament
☞ The patella
☞ The patellar tendon (ligamentum patellae)
☞ The adductor tubercle
☞ The head of the fibula
☞ The tendon of biceps femoris
☞ There is a popliteal pulse behind the knee – it is not always easy to find, flex your model's knee to 45° and see if it is palpable.

Ligament tests in the knee joint

If your model has a known knee problem consult your lecturer before doing the tests below. There are many tests but these are the most important ones. You must be able to demonstrate the following tests:

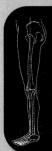

☞ AP draw = PCL
☞ PA draw = ACL
☞ Varus stress test = LCL
☞ Valgus stress test = MCL.

☞ Test the integrity of your model's medial collateral ligament. Why flex the knee slightly?

Your notes

☞ Test the integrity of your model's lateral collateral ligament. Why flex the knee slightly?

Your notes

☞ Test the integrity of your model's anterior cruciate ligament.

Your notes

☞ Test the integrity of your model's posterior cruciate ligament.

Your notes

What would be the significance of the following when these tests are carried out:

1 Pain?

2 Excessive movement?

3 Refusal by the patient?

☞ What movements are possible at the knee joint?
☞ Ask your model to perform them and carefully observe the muscles contracting.
☞ A fellow student is arguing with you; he says that the knee is a hinge joint. How do you convince him that he is wrong?
☞ What is conjunct rotation?
☞ What bony points can be palpated around the knee?

List them below.

☞ Ask your model to lie down. Move your model's patella – in how many directions can it be moved?
☞ Can the model do this voluntarily?
☞ What is the term for this type of movement?
☞ Now repeat, after asking your model to contract their quadriceps muscle – what do you notice?

☞ Why is this an important fact for your future career?
☞ What is the function of the patella?

Clue: The patella is *not* a shock absorber, if it were, there would be patellae all over the body!

The menisci

13 ☞ What is the function of the menisci?

☞ How many are there in each knee?

☞ Draw the menisci below.

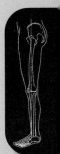

from above   in cross section

☞ What are the differences between medial and lateral menisci?

☞ Why do you need to know this?

☞ Draw below two ways in which menisci might tear.

PROFESSOR ASKS

☞ Are the menisci palpable?
☞ How are the menisci anchored to the tibia?
☞ Why does the hip joint not require menisci?

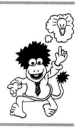

14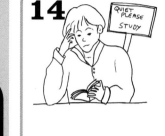

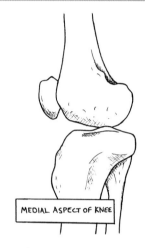

MEDIAL ASPECT OF KNEE

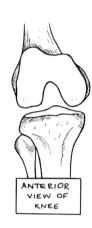

ANTERIOR VIEW OF KNEE

To the above diagrams, add the:

❑ cruciate ligaments × 2
❑ collateral ligaments × 2
❑ menisci × 2
❑ Where would a fabella be?
❑ Draw it on the diagram
❑ What is a sesamoid bone?

Answers

☞ The anterior margin may be palpated.
☞ Coronary ligaments.
☞ Bones themselves are congruent unlike the knee joint.

The superior tibiofibular joint

Surface marking and joint line

Bones involved

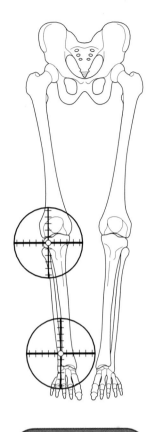

Joint classification

Ligaments

Movements possible

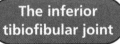

The inferior tibiofibular joint

Surface marking and joint line

Bones involved

Joint classification

Ligaments

Movements possible – some gapping occurs to permit final degrees of ankle dorsiflexion.

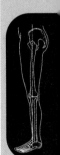

15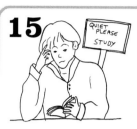

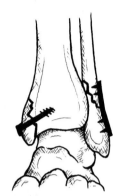

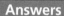

Look at this problem.

I want you to understand that we make you study all this anatomy for a reason. Fred broke his ankle 6 months ago; the fracture was fixed surgically by placing a metal plate on the sides of his lower tibia and fibula (internal fixation). The fracture is now healed. The picture below shows you how the fracture has been fixed.

He comes to see you and is complaining that he cannot 'pull his foot up' (dorsiflex the ankle joint). (He has lost the final 5° of dorsiflexion when you measure his movements.)

- Using what you have learned about the tibiofibular joint so far, think of why this might be so.
- Why has the medial malleolus been screwed back in place?
- What would happen to the ankle joint if this had not been done?
- What is an ORIF?

Answers

- Final degrees of dorsiflexion are achieved by gapping of inferior tibfib joint.
- Medial malleolus needs accurate reduction – reduction means aligning the bone ends after a fracture as it forms part of the ankle joint mortice.
- Failure to fix this might result in an unstable ankle joint in the future and secondary osteoarthritis.
- Open reduction internal fixation.

16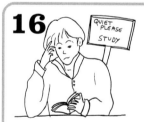

- How does the knee joint maintain its stability yet it is able to move through a wide range of motion?

  Time yourself – 15 minutes to answer.

- How is the structure of the knee joint related to its function?

  Write a whole page of A4 on this.

Answer tips

If you are asked a question like this, do not just describe the structure and then describe the function – that is probably the commonest way to fail this type of question. Instead, link the two, e.g. the knee joint is a very mobile joint which is extended by the quadriceps muscle group – potentially at a mechanical disadvantage since it approaches the tibial tuberosity almost parallel to the femoral shaft. To minimise

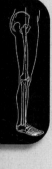

this, the knee joint has a patella to achieve a more efficient extension mechanism, changing the angle of approach of the quadriceps tendon.

Your turn!

THE ANKLE JOINT

Hold an articulated (joined) foot in your hand. Look at the superior surface of the talus: it is wedge shaped, fatter anteriorly, narrower posteriorly. This is relevant because it means that when the ankle is plantarflexed, the narrow part of the talus is in contact with the malleoli, allowing a large gap on either side and therefore more movement. When dorsiflexed, the wide part of the talus is locked between the malleoli, making it stable with almost no movement available, in fact the final few degrees of dorsiflexion are achieved by gapping apart of the tibia and fibula.

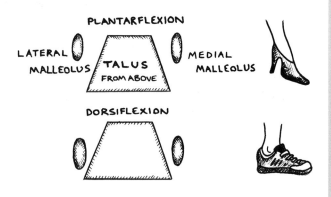

PLANTARFLEXION

LATERAL MALLEOLUS TALUS FROM ABOVE MEDIAL MALLEOLUS

DORSIFLEXION

Medial.

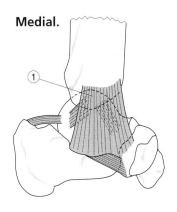

The collateral ligaments of the ankle joint

Therefore the closed packed position for the ankle is full dorsiflexion. The ankle is therefore less stable in plantarflexion and most injuries to the ligaments of the ankle occur when the foot is in some degree of plantar flexion (stiletto wearers beware!), e.g. when walking *down* stairs.

Lateral.

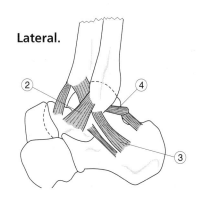

Joints of the lower limb

Summary – medial and lateral ligaments of the ankle joint:

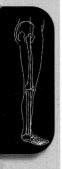

1 Deltoid	2 Anterior talo fibular	3 Calcaneo fibular	4 Posterior talo fibular
Name	Name	Name	Name
Attachments	Attachments	Attachments	Attachments
Function	Function	Function	Function

Think about it, it makes perfect sense to put strong ligaments on either side of a hinge joint – if they were at the front and back they would interfere with movement and not resist lateral forces. Millions of years of evolution has done a pretty good job of preparing us for the stresses and strains which the body will have to endure.

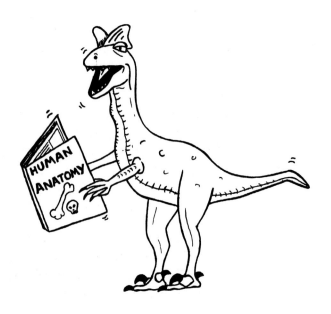

Remembering the lateral collateral ligamens at the ankle

Slide your hand down the outside of your leg, this more or less corresponds to the three lateral ligaments at the ankle joint.

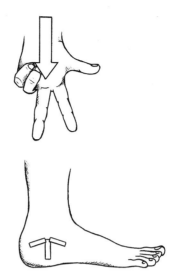

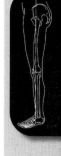

PROFESSOR ASKS

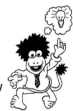

So, why does the hip joint not have two collateral ligaments?

You haven't done it yet but if I told you that the elbow was a hinge joint, where would you put two ligaments?

17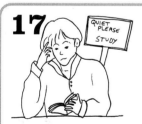

☞ List the differences between medial and lateral collateral ligaments at the ankle.
☞ What is an avulsion fracture?
☞ Why are avulsion fractures common at the medial malleolus and not the lateral malleolus?
☞ What does collateral mean?

Answers

☞ Look it up!
☞ Detachment of a piece of bone as a result of pull of associated ligament or tendon.
☞ Deltoid ligament is very strong and so may pull off the tip of the medial malleolus unlike the lateral ligament which will rupture first.
☞ Collateral means either side.

☞ The surface marking of the ankle joint =
☞ The surface marking of the subtalar joint =
☞ The surface marking of the midtarsal joint =

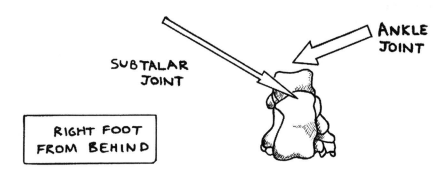

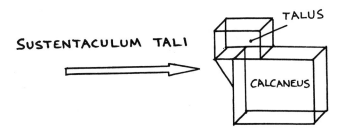

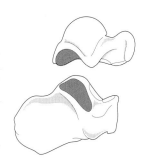

This is where things get complicated (if they weren't already).

The ankle joint (talocrural joint) is between the tibia/fibula and the superior surface of the talus it is a hinge joint allowing dorsi and plantarflexion.

The talus sits on top of the calcaneus but not completely, so the calcaneus needs a scaffolding to *sustain* or hold the talus up. This is called the sustentaculum tali.

There is a joint on the underside of the talus between this and the superior surface of the calcaneus – the subtalar (talocalcanean) joint.

There are two points of contact here, anterior and posterior.

THE SUBTALAR JOINT

The joint has a concave posterior facet on inferior surface of talus and the convex posterior facet on the upper surface of the calcaneus.

Movements at subtalar level (complicated)

Movement at the subtalar joint is often described as inversion and eversion. The triplanar motion of the talus occurs around a single axis, allowing components of pronation and supination to occur.

Think of the surfaces of the subtalar joint forming a cylinder whose long axis passes obliquely through the sinus tarsi.

The axis of the subtalar joint

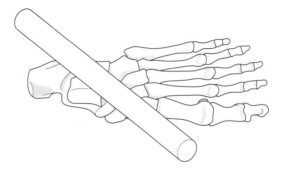

Supination is calcaneal inversion + adduction + plantarflexion. **Pronation** is abduction calcaneal eversion + dorsiflexion (remember prone to <u>bed</u> = <u>ab</u>duction <u>E</u>version <u>D</u>orsiflexion). Note that these movements all occur together and cannot be separated. Much gliding and rotation occurs at these two joints, by which the foot rotates underneath the talus. Inversion and eversion occur here. The axis for movement runs forwards, upwards and medially from the back of the calcaneus, through the sinus tarsi to emerge at the superomedial aspect of the neck of the talus.

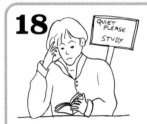

18 **Describe the subtalar joint.**

- The bones involved.
- How they articulate.
- The ligaments involved

  – Lateral talocalcanean
  – Medial talocalcanean
  – Interosseous talocalcanean
  – Cervical
  – The axis of motion.

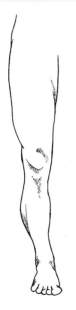

Draw on each other and on this diagram:

- ❏ Greater trochanter
- ❏ Head of fibula
- ❏ Tendon of biceps femoris
- ❏ Lateral collateral ligament of the knee
- ❏ Tensor fascia latae
- ❏ Lateral malleolus
- ❏ Peroneus longus
- ❏ Peroneus brevis
- ❏ Tubercle at base of 5th metatarsal.

Clue

Draw the lateral ligaments of the ankle on this picture and on your model.

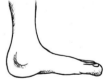

Draw the medial ligament (deltoid) of the ankle on this picture and on your model.

Clue

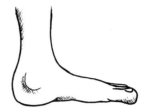

On this diagram and on your model, draw the:

❑ Medial and lateral heads of gastrocnemius
❑ The musculotendinous junction
❑ Soleus
❑ The Achilles tendon
❑ Tibialis anterior.

To this posterior view, add the bones which make up the ankle joint.

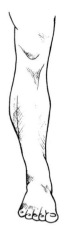

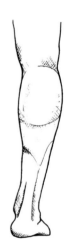

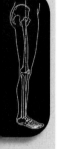

The ankle – practical

✍ On your model, draw the malleoli.
✍ Add the collateral ligaments.
✍ Dorsiflex your ankle and identify as many tendons as you can.
✍ Repeat and draw them on the leg of your model as they contract.
✍ Draw on your model the deltoid and lateral ligaments of the ankle.
✍ Draw on your model the retinaculae.
✍ What does retinaculum mean? What is their function?
✍ Draw on your model the plantar fascia – with care if they are ticklish.
✍ Draw the cuboid, tuberosity of navicular, neck of the talus, base of 5th metatarsal bone on your model.
✍ Draw the MTP joints, the IP joints and the head of the fibula on your model.
✍ Find the anterior tibial, dorsalis pedis and posterior tibial pulses on your model.

On your model, label the following:

    ☞ Malleoli
    ☞ The tendons of extensor digitorum longus
    ☞ The tendons of extensor digitorum brevis
    ☞ Extensor hallucis longus
    ☞ The retinaculae
    ☞ Tendon of tibialis anterior.

If you are unsure about which tendon is which, ask your model to stand on one leg, their extensor tendons/dorsiflexors, etc., will work like crazy, especially if you make the model work by, for example, catching a ball.

On the diagrams and then on the leg of your model, draw the following:

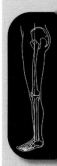

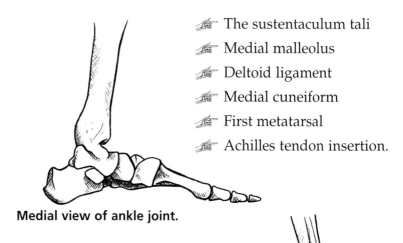

    ☞ The sustentaculum tali
    ☞ Medial malleolus
    ☞ Deltoid ligament
    ☞ Medial cuneiform
    ☞ First metatarsal
    ☞ Achilles tendon insertion.

Medial view of ankle joint.

    ☞ Lateral malleolus
    ☞ The three lateral collateral ligaments
    ☞ The cuboid bone
    ☞ Tuberosity at the base of
       the 5th metatarsal.

Lateral view of ankle joint.

Making it real

Anatomy should not be thought of as a text-book subject. It is probably the basis for the rest of your careers. I would like you to take a moment to think about why I ask you to learn anatomy in such great detail.

Try these problems …

1 A patient comes to see you. He felt a 'twang' in the back of his leg yesterday when he was running to catch the bus. Passive SLR (straight leg raise) produces posterior thigh pain and so does resisted knee flexion, this is made worse by resisted lateral rotation of the knee.

- ❑ Which muscle has he damaged?
- ❑ How do you know?
- ❑ What led you to your conclusion?

2 After a night clubbing you 'go over' on your ankle; you have forcibly inverted your ankle joint walking down some stairs:

- ❑ Which ligaments have been stressed?
- ❑ Which is the likeliest ligament to be damaged?
- ❑ Why would this probably not have happened walking up stairs?

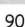

3 A friend stops you in the street. He has noticed a pain on the lateral side of his hip region following a long walk; he can feel a click when he swings his leg forwards and his leg aches around the greater trochanter area but he can move his hip fully with no pain. He is convinced that his hip is 'coming out of its socket'.

From your knowledge of anatomy:

- ❑ How can you be confident that this is unlikely?
- ❑ What could be happening?
- ❑ Is it relatively easy or hard to dislocate a hip joint? (not a hip replacement)

Answers 1

☞ Biceps femoris.
☞ Work it out – read Chapter 3.
☞ All resisted actions of the muscle are painful.

Answers 2

☞ Lateral ligament complex.
☞ Anterior talofibular ligament.
☞ Dorsiflexed ankle = close packed = more stable.

Answers 3

☞ It is very difficult to dislocate a healthy hip joint, it takes major trauma to do so, a car crash for example.
☞ What could be happening is ilio-tibial band syndrome, caused by overuse or inflamation of the ilio tibial band.
☞ Very difficult – go and watch a hip replacement!

Talocalcaneonav-icular joint (TCN)

This joint is between the ovoid head of the talus and concave posterior of the navicular, and the middle and anterior facets of the talus on the calcaneus. The spring ligament (plantar calcaneonavicular) also contributes to this complex joint. Together with the calcaneocuboid joint these two joints form the junction between hindfoot and midfoot.

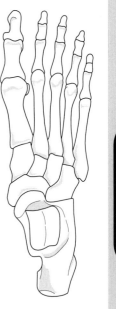

The calcaneocuboid joint

Your notes

The cuneonavicular joint

Your notes

The cuboidonav-icular joint

Your notes

The tarsometa-tarsal joints

Your notes

Joints of the lower limb

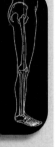

The intermeta-tarsal joints

Your notes

The metatar-sophalangeal joints

Your notes

The interpha-langeal joints

Your notes

Joints of the foot – a brief summary.

- THE ANKLE (TALOCRURAL) JOINT

= HINGE JOINT

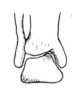

- SUBTALAR (TALOCALCANEAL) JOINT COMPLEX, OBLIQUE AXIS

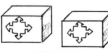

- INTERTARSAL JOINTS

PLANE JOINTS, A SMALL AMOUNT OF GLIDING OCCURS HERE

19 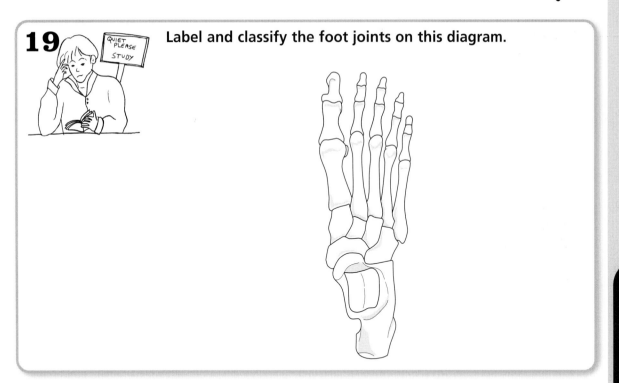 **Label and classify the foot joints on this diagram.**

Here, I have separated the bones of the foot so that you can add your own notes on the joints if you wish.

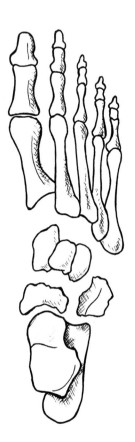

20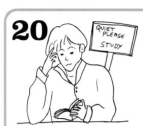

The plantar fascia:

Where is it?

What is its function?

What are its attachments?

The arches of the foot:

List them

Describe their structure

How are they maintained?

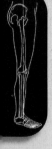

21

The retinaculae of the leg:

Where are they?

What is their function?

What are their attachments?

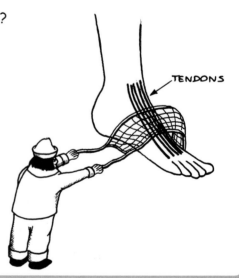

TENDONS

Long and short plantar ligaments:

Where are they?

What is their function?

What are their attachments?

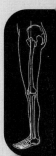

LIMITING FACTORS

The soft tissue parts of a joint that may limit movement ligament, capsule, tendon, muscle, meniscus.

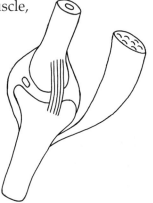

Bone to bone contact may limit movement – elbow extension, for example.

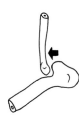

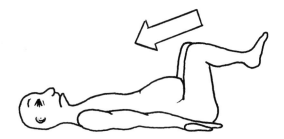

Unfortunately, sometimes our soft tissues get in the way, e.g. hip flexion.

You need to know what *should* limit movement in a normal joint before you can tell what is abnormal.

Joint	Limiting factors (normal joint)
Hip	
Flexion	Soft tissue (abdomen!)
Extension	Iliofemoral ligament + hip flexors
Medial rotation	Lateral rotators, posterior capsule, ischiofemoral ligament
Lateral rotation	Medial rotators, lateral band iliofemoral ligament
Abduction	Adductors medial band iliofemoral ligament
Adduction	Abductors, ligamentum teres, lateral band iliofemoral ligament
Knee	
Extension	Both collaterals, posterior capsule, skin, fascia, hamstrings, gastrocnemius, parts of both cruciates, anterior menisci (squeezed)
Flexion	Parts of both cruciates, posterior menisci (squeezed), quadriceps, anterior capsule soft tissue approximation
Ankle	
Dorsiflexion	Achilles tendon (if knee is extended) Posterior deltoid ligament Calcaneofibular ligament
Plantarflexion	By dorsiflexors Anterior deltoid ligament Anterior talofibular ligament

Before your written and practical examinations, go through each of these points, can you write about each in detail and demonstrate it practically?

Joints

You should be able to identify practically on a model and write about in detail for written exams:

Hip

- ❏ Joint line
- ❏ Movements
- ❏ Limiting factors to movement
- ❏ Bones involved
- ❏ Classification
- ❏ Three capsular ligaments/ligamentum teres.

Knee

- ❏ Joint line
- ❏ Movements
- ❏ Limiting factors to movement
- ❏ Bones involved
- ❏ Classification

- ❑ Anterior and posterior cruciate ligaments
- ❑ Medial and lateral collateral ligaments
- ❑ Other ligaments less important, e.g. transverse, arcuate popliteal ligament, etc.

Patellofemoral joint and superior and inferior tibiofibular joints

- ❑ Palpate location
- ❑ Joint line
- ❑ Classification
- ❑ Ligaments.

Ankle

- ❑ Joint line
- ❑ Movements
- ❑ Limiting factors to movement
- ❑ Bones involved
- ❑ Classification
- ❑ Three lateral ligaments
- ❑ Medial (deltoid) ligament.

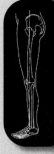

Subtalar

- ❑ Movements
- ❑ Limiting factors to movement
- ❑ Bones involved
- ❑ Classification
- ❑ Ligaments.

Intertarsal and tarsometatarsal joints

(Less detail needed)

- ❑ Bones involved
- ❑ Classification
- ❑ Movements possible
- ❑ Main ligaments.

Metatarso-phalangeal and interpalangeal joints

- ❑ Bones involved
- ❑ Classification
- ❑ Movements possible
- ❑ Main ligaments.

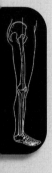

Judgement time

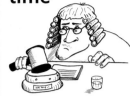

It is now time for you to assess whether or not you have achieved the learning outcomes at the start of this chapter. You need to be able to tick each of these boxes, if you cannot, return to the relevant section of the chapter.

❑ Can you describe (for your written paper and orally for your exams) the structure of all joints of the lower limb including articular surfaces, movements possible, ligaments, capsule and other important features particular to that joint?

❑ Can you describe (for your written paper and orally for your exams) the function of all joints of the lower limb?

❑ Could you relate 1 (above) to 2 (above)?

❑ Do you have a working knowledge of limiting factors to movements of the joints of the lower limb?

❑ Are you able to demonstrate surface marking of hip, knee, ankle, subtalar and midtarsal joints?

MUSCLES OF THE LOWER LIMB

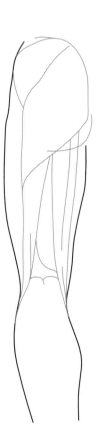

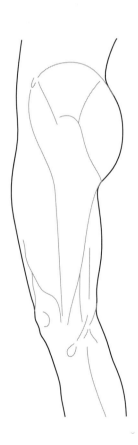

Muscles of the lower limb

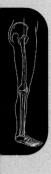

WHAT THIS CHAPTER IS

A chapter introducing the muscles of the lower limb. It attempts to put things across in a simple way using as many tricks, rhymes and so on as I can think of. This covers or tells you what <u>you</u> need to cover in order for you to gain maximum benefit from the classroom sessions. I have designed it to enhance the lectures in class and encourage <u>you</u> to undertake self directed study.

LEARNING OUTCOMES

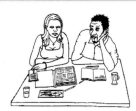

In this chapter and the relevant lectures and practical sessions you should be able to describe in writing and verbally the:

1 Origin
2 Insertion
3 Action
4 Functional (applied) anatomy
5 Nerve supply

of the muscles contained in this chapter.

Learn these terms and don't argue!

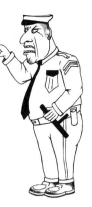

- ☞ **Concentric:** muscle contraction which results in the muscle becoming shorter.
- ☞ **Eccentric:** when a muscle gradually controls movement by slowly lengthening – paying out length. Actin and myosin overlap decreases.
- ☞ **Isometric:** when there is no change in muscle length, e.g. a bodybuilder posing. Sarcomere length is constant.
- ☞ **Reciprocal lengthening:** as a set of muscles work concentrically, the opposite muscles have to lengthen to allow movement otherwise we would never move anywhere!
- ☞ **Reciprocal shortening:** as a set of muscles work eccentrically, the opposite muscles have to 'gather up the slack' but the muscle is not actively contracting. There is some cross-bridge formation.

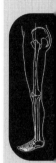

> Concentric . . . eccentric . . . What's that all about then?

This is a tricky concept. Once you grasp it it's not that hard but until you do it will cause you some problems.

Here is my attempt to explain it.

Imagine a crane that has to lift a heavy weight. It does this by attaching a rope to it and winching up the rope. To lower the weight it still uses the same rope but the rope slowly pays out its length and gently lowers the weight to the floor.

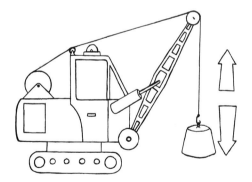

As the rope shortens the weight is pulled up = concentric contraction.

As the rope lengthens the weight is gently lowered = eccentric contraction.

MUSCLES AROUND THE HIP JOINT

Because the hip joint is multi-axial joint (it can move in lots of directions), it needs many muscle groups to achieve and control movement. If it were a hinge joint it would only need flexors and extensors and your student life would be a lot simpler. In reality though these are the groups of muscles that act at the hip joint.

Muscles of the lower limb

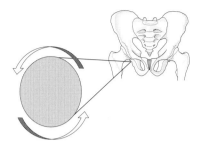

- ☞ Flexors
- ☞ Extensors
- ☞ Abductors
- ☞ Adductors
- ☞ Lateral rotators
- ☞ Medial rotators.

All the above work in combination to produce circumduction – where the foot would trace out a cone.

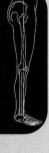

Hip flexors   Complete this table

Muscle	Action	Origin	Insertion	Nerve supply
Psoas major	Hip flexion			
Psoas minor	Hip flexion			
Iliacus	Hip flexion			
Rectus femoris	Hip flexion			
	Knee extension			
Sartorius	Hip flexion			
	Abduction			
	External rotation			
	Knee flexion			
	Knee internal rotation			

Psoas and iliacus are too deep to palpate. Sartorius is the body's longest muscle and although not often injured it is used in many movements, especially when sitting cross-legged (sartorial means to do with tailoring). To demonstrate its action, imagine you had stepped on a drawing pin or something nasty in the street, and look at the sole of your own foot – this is what sartorius does.

Test Yourself

On this picture, find the following muscles:

☞ Psoas major
☞ Iliacus.

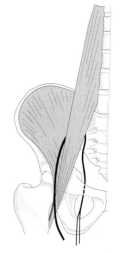
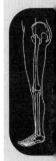

Iliacus + psoas are sometimes called the iliopsoas.

☞ It has the potential to stabilise the lumbar spine (Santaguida & McGill 1995).
☞ Muscle imbalance affecting the muscles of the hip joint is now thought to be a possible cause of low back pain (Nadler *et al*. 2001).

Hip extensors

Complete this table

Muscle	Action	Origin	Insertion	Nerve supply
Gluteus maximus				
Biceps femoris				
Semitendinosus				
Semimembranosus				

Gluteus maximus is the bulkiest muscle in the body.

It also helps to control knee stability – how does it do this?

Clue: only some of its fibres attach to the femur.

Muscles of the lower limb

Answer 75% of its fibres attach to the iliotibial band which crosses the knee joint and therefore can have a stabilising effect on it.

Hip abductors Complete this table

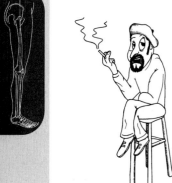

Muscle	Action	Origin	Insertion	Nerve supply
Gluteus minimus				
Gluteus medius				
Tensor fascia latae				

How to remember the hip abductors/medial rotators

Tensor fascia latae, gluteus med & min, all abduct the femur, and rotate it in.

Hip adductors Complete this table

Muscle	Action	Origin	Insertion	Nerve supply
Adductor longus				
Adductor brevis				
Adductor magnus				
Pectineus				
Gracilis				

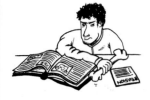

How to remember: **3 ducks peck** at the **grass**
(hip adductors = 3 ad**duc**tors, **pec**tineus and **gra**cilis).

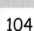

Label the hip adductors on this picture
(colour them in if it helps).

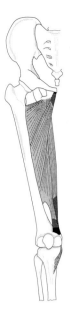

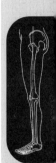

A typical anatomy viva question: what movement do the hip
adductors limit?
(Answer = abduction.)

**Hip lateral
rotators**

Complete this table

Muscle	Action	Origin	Insertion	Nerve supply
Quadratus femoris				
Piriformis				
Obturator internus				
Obturator externus				
Gemellus superior				
Gemellus inferior				

These six muscles are all too deep to palpate. They are rarely injured
so I don't want you to spend long hours worrying about them.

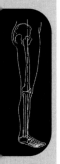

Hip medial rotators

Complete this table

Muscle	Action	Origin	Insertion	Nerve supply
Tensor fascia latae				
Gluteus medius				
Gluteus minimus				

See your previous notes on these muscles. The medial rotators also abduct the hip – saves you some revision at least!

Psoas and iliacus are stretched during lying prone.

Normal iliopsoas.

Flexion contracture.

If there are soft tissue contractures in these muscles or the anterior of the hip capsule, lying or prone lying is painful or impossible – see Thomas test.

Most patients with chronic back pain find lying flat uncomfortable because psoas also attaches to the lumbar spine and pulls on this spinal attachment in lying.

Gluteus maximus works hard when rising from a sitting position and extending the hip joint during push off phase of walking. If you have a patient on long-term bed rest, don't forget that these muscles atrophy (weaken) very quickly.

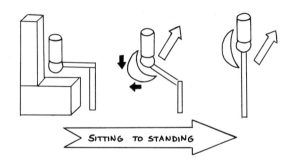

SITTING TO STANDING

> The hip abductors abduct the hip – no surprise there!

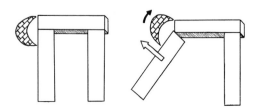

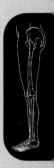

But – did you know that they also prevent adduction of the hip and prevent the pelvis from falling when standing on the same leg? If they are too weak to do this, the pelvis drops – see Trendelenberg sign.

You could think of the pelvis as a plank balanced on top of a golf ball (femoral head). The plank can tip either way, the hip abductors help control the plank!

THE GLUTEAL GREMLIN

The Trendelenberg sign is quite a difficult concept to grasp, so here goes with a really silly demonstration. I don't care that it is silly as long as it helps you to work it out. If it does not, please do not think any less of me, I'll be OK!

First of all imagine that the picture below represents the pelvis and hip joint.

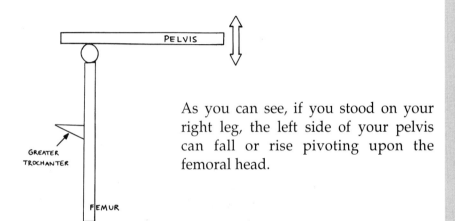

PELVIS

GREATER TROCHANTER

FEMUR

As you can see, if you stood on your right leg, the left side of your pelvis can fall or rise pivoting upon the femoral head.

Now meet Gerald who will act out the role of gluteus medius and minimus for this demonstration.

See if this little guy helps you to understand the role of the hip abductors in maintaining a level pelvis.

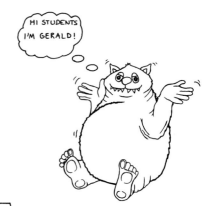

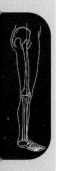

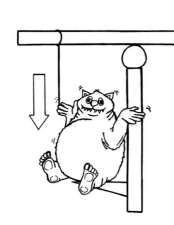

Gerald is the Gluteal Gremlin. He has a rope in his hand and his bottom is glued to the greater trochanter. Because he is so strong, he pulls on the rope and keeps the weight level.

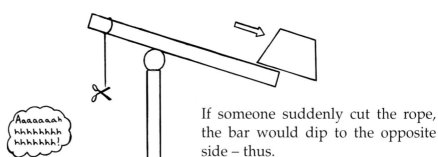

If someone suddenly cut the rope, the bar would dip to the opposite side – thus.

This is what happens when the hip abductor muscles are weak. They allow the opposite side of the pelvis to dip.

HUNG UP ON ACTIONS/ORIGINS AND INSERTIONS?

Do not forget that whilst a muscle has an action, e.g. flexion, it also resists the opposite movement. For example, biceps flexes the elbow but it can also prevent elbow extension, the hip abductors abduct the hip but they can also prevent adduction.

So what? Just because the anatomy books say that a muscle is an abductor, doesn't mean that all day long it abducts and does nothing else. How often do you actually abduct your hip during the course of a normal day? It is far more likely that you will use the abductors to prevent adduction as shown above. Never forget that functional anatomy is extremely important, i.e. how things actually work in a living body.

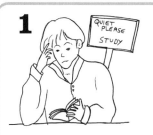

1 **Imagine that you have been set the following exam question:**

Give a detailed account of the muscles that abduct the hip joint and explain the signs and symptoms that would result from weakness of these muscles, and state how weakness of these muscles can be assessed clinically.

Answer on a page.

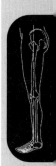

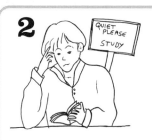

2 The other important test that you need to understand at the hip is the Thomas test. This is a test for a hip flexion deformity. Make notes below on:

☞ How to perform the test
☞ What the test demonstrates
☞ What a positive result looks like
☞ You could be asked to demonstrate this in your practical exam.

Note that the Thomas test does not test for the *strength* of the hip flexors – it is a test of their *length*. *Students often get this confused.*

GLUTEUS MAXIMUS – PRACTICAL

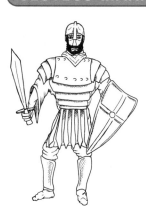

And no, gluteus maximus was not a Roman general or a gladiator!

☞ Find the muscle on this picture and then draw it on your partner.
☞ In which direction do its fibres run?
☞ Demonstrate its functional activity.
☞ What are its origins and insertions?

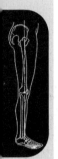

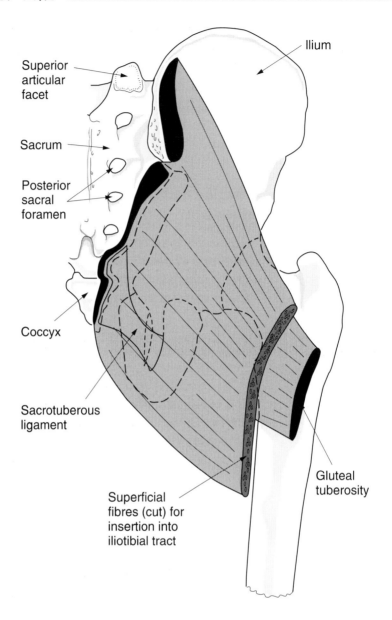

Superior articular facet

Ilium

Sacrum

Posterior sacral foramen

Coccyx

Sacrotuberous ligament

Superficial fibres (cut) for insertion into iliotibial tract

Gluteal tuberosity

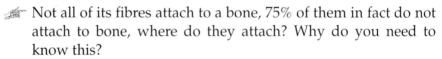

- Not all of its fibres attach to a bone, 75% of them in fact do not attach to bone, where do they attach? Why do you need to know this?
- Why do injections in this muscle have to be carefully placed?
- *Clue:* what nerve passes deep to this muscle?
- Is it possible to palpate the following?

  ❑ obturator internus
  ❑ obturator externus
  ❑ gemellus inferior
  ❑ gemellus superior
  ❑ quadratus femoris
  ❑ piriformis.

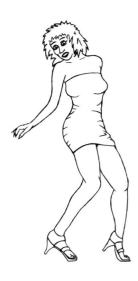

☞ Think of an everyday activity involving hip extension for which gluteus maximus is needed.

☞ Think of a type of patient who might need exercises to strengthen a weak gluteus maximus.

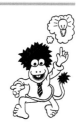

PROFESSOR'S TIP OF THE DAY

You would think that a big sounding muscle would be supplied by a big sounding nerve right? Well think again – gluteus **maximus** is supplied by the **inferior** gluteal nerve (remember a model thinking his or her **bottom** is **inferior**).

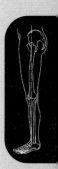

HIP ABDUCTORS – PRACTICAL

☞ How would a person walk if the hip abduction were weak?

☞ Demonstrate the gait to your partner.

☞ These two muscles insert onto the greater trochanter, so how can a forensic pathologist determine whether a skeleton belonged to a body-builder or a couch potato by looking at a greater trochanter and other bony lumps and bumps?

☞ Apart from hip abduction, what is the function of the hip abductors?

☞ Is there a difference between medial and internal rotation?

☞ Is there a difference between external and lateral rotation?

☞ You are chatting to a patient who has had a total hip replacement. Their surgical incision goes through the gluteus medius and minimus – the patient is very concerned that when they walk, their operation leg tends to roll into external rotation and it is difficult for them to correct this. How do you explain this to your patient using your knowledge of anatomy?

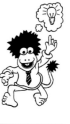

PROFESSOR'S TIP OF THE DAY

To palpate gluteus medius and minimus, stand with your legs slightly apart, place your hand above your greater trochanter but below your iliac crest, rock gently from side to side or stand on one leg – they contract strongly on the weight-bearing leg.

Muscles of the lower limb

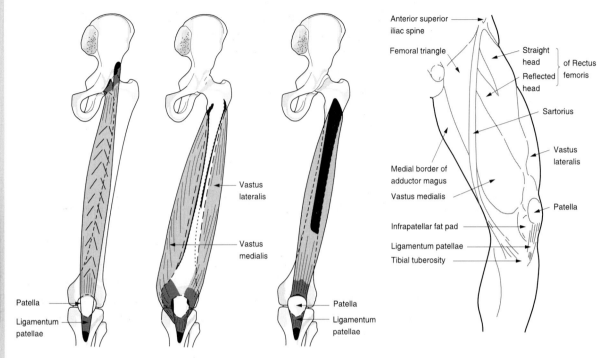
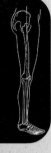

Vastus
lateralis

Vastus
medialis

Patella

Ligamentum
patellae

Patella

Ligamentum
patellae

Anterior superior
iliac spine

Femoral triangle

Straight
head
Reflected
head
} of Rectus
femoris

Sartorius

Vastus
lateralis

Medial border of
adductor magus

Vastus medialis

Patella

Infrapatellar fat pad

Ligamentum patellae

Tibial tuberosity

1 What does 'ceps' mean?
2 What does 'quad' mean?
3 List the component muscles of the quadriceps group below.

(i)

(ii)

(iii)

(iv)

4 Which is the odd one out and why?
5 Which one is too deep to palpate?
6 How does the patella ensure that the quadriceps can work effectively?

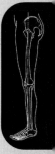

Answers

1 Head.
2 Four.
3 Vastus intermedius, lateralis, medialis rectus femoris.
4 Rectus femoris because it acts across the hip joint
   or v medialis because of its oblique pull
   or intermedius because of its depth
   or lateralis because it has a letter L!
5 Intermedius.
6 Changes the angle of approach of the patellar tendon.

THE Q ANGLE

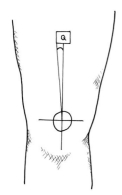

Exam tip – do not call them 'Quads' in exams and never use abbreviations unless you first define them.

On your model, draw a straight line across the middle of the patella. From the centre of this, draw a straight line going downwards through the centre of the tibial tuberosity, and another going upwards towards the ASIS.

Measure this angle using a goniometer.

This is known as the Q angle. It should be no more than 13° in males and no more than 18° in females – you will study this more in biomechanics.

Knowledge of this angle can assist with the diagnosis of patella maltracking.

THE HAMSTRINGS – PRACTICAL

Find the hamstrings on this diagram.

☞ How many hamstrings are there on each leg?
   Answer. 3

☞ On your model trace them from origin to insertion if possible. Why might this be difficult to do?

☞ Ask your model to lie prone and flex their knee to a right angle, then ask them to internally and externally rotate their leg.

☞ Which muscles are contracting during each part of the movement?

☞ If you have no spinal problems try this.

   ❑ Sit with your knees extended (long sitting)
   ❑ Try to touch your toes keeping your knees extended

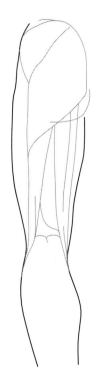

❏ Now repeat this with your knees flexed

❏ Why is it possible to go further if you flex your knees?

Answer. Muscles can stretch across one joint not two simultaneously.

☞ What is the term for this phenomenon?
Answer. Passive insufficiency – the inability of a muscle to stretch maximally simultaneously across two joints

☞ Why are the hamstrings often injured?
Answer. They are two joint muscles.

☞ What is the action of the hamstrings at:

(i) The hip joint?
Answer. Extension (lies posterior to joint axis).

(ii) The knee joint?
Answer. Flexion (lies posterior to joint axis).

(iii) How do the hamstrings manage to perform rotation at the knee joint?
Answer. They attach on either side of the posterior aspect of the knee and thus have a rotary component.

SARTORIUS – PRACTICAL

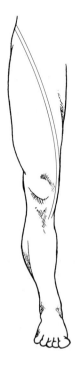

Think about the sartorius muscle.

☞ What is the action of this long, strap-like muscle?
Answer. Hip flexion abduction lateral rotation.

☞ How can you get your model to demonstrate sartorius at work?
Answer. Tell them they have just stepped on something smelly and wait till they look at the sole of their shoe!

☞ What does sartorial mean?
Answer. To do with tailoring. Apparently tailors used to sit cross-legged.

☞ On this diagram, then on your model, colour in:

❏ Sartorius
❏ Vastus medialis
❏ Rectus femoris
❏ Patellar tendon
❏ Tensor fascia latae

❏ The iliac crest
❏ The inguinal ligament.

☞ To find the femoral pulse, find the inguinal ligament, find its mid point and palpate just inferior to this.

☞ Find the pulse on three different models.

THE HIP ADDUCTORS – PRACTICAL

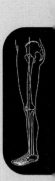

☞ On the inner (medial) thigh carefully find the tendon of adductor longus, the bellies of the adductors and the adductor tubercle.

☞ Ask your model to adduct against resistance and see which tendons can be palpated.

☞ Which of the hip adductors cross the knee joint?
Answer. Gracilis

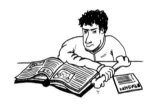

☞ Why do you need to know this?
Answer. If it crosses the joint it might have an effect on its stability so don't forget it when you are treating knees!

How do I remember the names of the hip adductors?

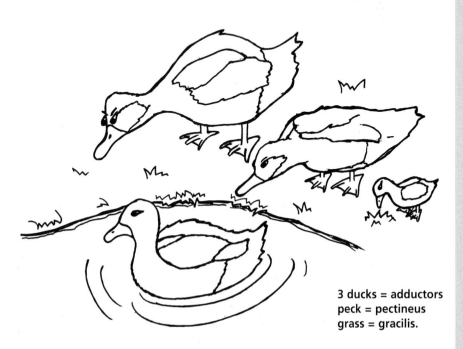

3 ducks = adductors
peck = pectineus
grass = gracilis.

Three ducks peck at the grass (please note that there is no grass though – they were really hungry!).

Muscles of the lower limb

Two theories as to why I have drawn three ducks pecking at some grass:

1 I am working too hard and probably starting to lose it!
2 It is a good trick to help you to remember the names and numbers of the adductors of the hip joint.

Label the three adductors, pectineus and gracilis; colour them in if it will help.

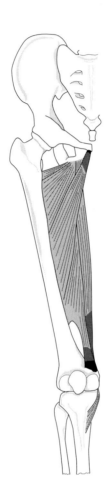

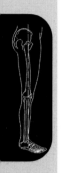

MUSCLES AROUND THE KNEE JOINT

These are:

☞ Flexors
☞ Extensors
☞ Lateral rotators
☞ Medial rotators.

There are others which cross the knee joint (therefore helping to stabilise it).

Knee flexors

Complete this table

Muscle	Action	Origin	Insertion	Nerve supply
Biceps femoris (2 heads)				
Semi-membranosus				
Semitendinosus				
Popliteus*				
Plantaris				
Gastrocnemius (2 heads)				

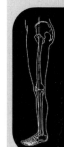

*Popliteus – the coolest muscle in the world! Popliteus is small but does some great things:

1 It unlocks the knee from full extension (remember we said that the knee was not a hinge joint – popliteus proves that. Without a popliteus you could not unlock your knees – imagine that!
2 It pulls the lateral meniscus out of the way during knee flexion to protect it – bless it.
3 Its origin is inside the knee joint so if you ever get chance to go and see an arthroscopy you may get to meet one in the flesh! (Incidentally my second choice for world's coolest muscle would be articularis genus – look it up in this book.)

The muscles that flex the knee joint

How can I remember the muscles that flex the knee?

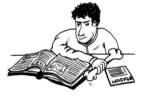

117

Muscles of the lower limb

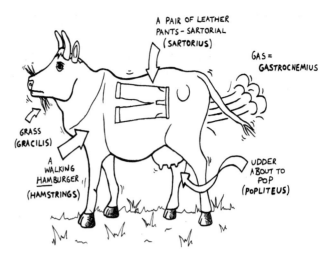

With thanks to Marc Hudson
1st year Physiotherapy student
(class of '99).

The muscles that flex the knee joint:

☞ Hamstrings*
☞ Gastrocnemius*
☞ Gracilis
☞ Sartorius
☞ Popliteus*
☞ *main role.

KNEE EXTENSORS

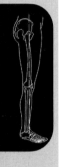

Complete this table

Muscle	Action	Origin	Insertion	Nerve supply
Rectus femoris				
Vastus intermedius				
Vastus lateralis				
Vastus medialis				
Articularis genus				

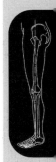

USELESS FACT NUMBER 356

There is a cute little muscle called articularis genus, which has been shown to have a very important function to perform. 'It elevates the capsule and the synovial membrane of the knee joint and prevents them from being pinched during extension of the leg' (Ahmad 1975).

So what?

So in theory teaching a person with an immobilised knee joint (such as a plaster cast) to do isometric quadriceps contractions will maintain the mobility of the synovium of the knee – it might be worth throwing that in to a practical exam or clinical placement sometime! Not a lot of people know that – now you do.

Pull the other one

Athletes often damage rectus femoris by extending the hip while simultaneously flexing the knee, e.g. kicking. Two joint muscles are frequently injured.

Look at how vastus medialis pulls at a much more oblique angle than the other three 'quads' in an attempt to prevent the patella being pulled too laterally (see maltracking patella/chondromalacia/recurrent dislocation of patella).

Right knee – anterior view.

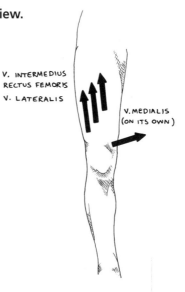

- V. INTERMEDIUS
- RECTUS FEMORIS
- V. LATERALIS

V. MEDIALIS (ON ITS OWN)

Question

There is another clever mechanism, which exists to prevent this tendency of the patella to be pulled laterally, what is it?

Answer

The lateral femoral condyle has a bony ridge to keep the patella in check, sometimes this is underdeveloped, leading to problems such as recurrent dislocations of the patella.

Muscles of the lower limb

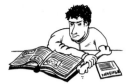

How to remember some important sites of muscle insertions.

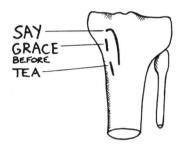

SAY —
GRACE
BEFORE
TEA —

S = SARTORIUS
G = GRACILIS
T = SEMITENDINOSUS

This rhyme may help you to remember the insertions of these three muscles. This region is sometimes called the pes anserinus, and the associated bursa the pes anserinus bursa.

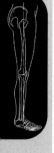

Injury to the hamstrings

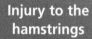

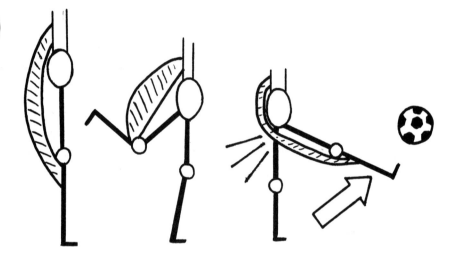

The hamstrings are posterior to the hip and knee joints so they flex the knee and extend the hip. If they are fully stretched over both hip and knee at the same time as in for example hurdling, or striking a football, they may tear. The inability to stretch across both joints at once is known as passive insufficiency.

MUSCLES AROUND THE ANKLE JOINT

These are

- Dorsiflexors
- Plantarflexors
- Invertors
- Evertors.

Ankle dorsiflexors

(*Note*: extrinsic muscles have origins in the leg but insertions in the foot.)

Tibialis anterior

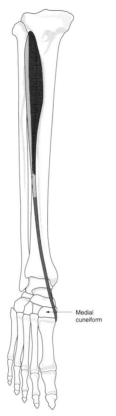

Medial cuneiform

Complete this table

Muscle	Action	Origin	Insertion	Nerve supply
Tibialis anterior				
Extensor hallucis longus				
Extensor digitorum longus				
Peroneus tertius (Not all people have one of these!)				

Tibialis anterior acts as a brake to decelerate the foot following heel strike in walking. If tibialis anterior is not working (e.g. after injury to the common peroneal nerve), a foot drop occurs, this may be heard as the foot slaps on the ground.

Ankle plantarflexors

Complete this table

Muscle	Action	Origin	Insertion	Nerve supply
Gastrocnemius				
Soleus (gastrocnemius and soleus together are sometimes referred to as the triceps surae)				
Tibialis posterior				
Plantaris (flexor hallucis longus) (flexor digitorum longus)				

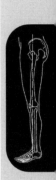

Gastrocnemius is mainly fast twitch, soleus is mainly slow twitch. What does this statement mean? Make sure you understand the differences between type I and type II muscle fibres.

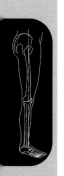

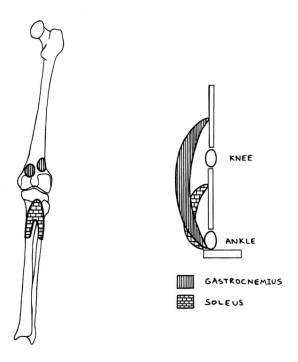

☞ What does gastrocnemius do that soleus does not?
Answer. Flexes the knee.

☞ Where does the Achilles tendon insert?
Answer. Look it up, don't get lazy on me.

☞ What is the triceps surae?
Answer. Old term for gastrocnemius and soleus combined – 'sural' refers to the leg.

☞ What is a fabella?
Answer. A small sesamoid bone embedded in one of the heads of gastrocnemius, not everyone has one and it can appear like a loose body on a lateral knee X-ray.

☞ How can one diagnose a ruptured Achilles tendon?
Answers. Squeeze test/Thompson test. Lie the patient prone with their foot over edge of the bed and squeeze their calf: no movement – ruptured tendon; slight plantarflexion – intact Achilles tendon. Once you know how – try the test on your model.

☞ What do you understand by the term musculotendinous (MT) junction?

☞ Draw the MT junctions of gastrocnemius on your model.

☞ On your model, draw the Achilles tendon.

More on gastrocnemius and soleus

On this diagram, label the following:

☞ Plantaris
☞ Soleus
☞ The Achilles tendon.

Gastrocnemius, soleus and plantaris.

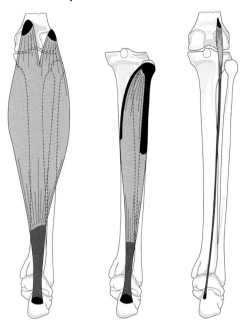
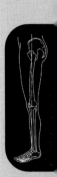

☞ On your model, demonstrate a functional activity of gastrocnemius and soleus
☞ Find peroneus longus and brevis
☞ Find the Achilles tendon.

Invertors

Complete this table

Muscle	Action	Origin	Insertion	Nerve supply
Tibialis anterior				
Tibialis posterior (FDL, FHL assist)				

Muscles of the lower limb

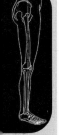

Evertors

Complete this table

Muscle	Action	Origin	Insertion	Nerve supply
Peroneus longus				
Peroneus brevis				
Peroneus tertius **Not everybody has one of these! It is sometimes considered as a 5th tendon of EDL**				

The peronei

These muscles often cause confusion amongst students. They are evertors of the foot and plantarflexors of the ankle.

Typical anatomy practical exam questions:

Q. Why do they evert the ankle?
A. Because they are on the lateral aspect of the leg.
Q. Why do they assist plantar flexion?
A. Because they pass behind the lateral malleolus and therefore are posterior to the ankle joint.

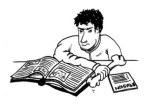

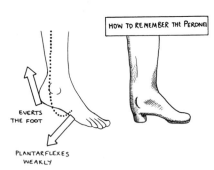

HOW TO REMEMBER THE PERONEI

EVERTS THE FOOT

PLANTARFLEXES WEAKLY

Imagine a pair of knee high boots
Sounds like per-o-ne-i
The zip on the outside of the boot corresponds to the location of the peronei.

Tip of the day

Students very often get mixed up between the muscles supplied by the deep and superficial peroneal nerves. Here are two alternative methods that will help, one for the boys, one for the girls!

GIRLS. You get back from the shops after having purchased your designer 'peroknee' high boots (above) and your flat-mate accuses you of being very superficial (thus you remember that the *peronei* are supplied by the *superficial* peroneal nerve).

BOYS. Your bank manager refuses you a loan so you stand face on to him and kick him in the *shins* causing a *deep* bruise (not that I advocate violence). Thus you remember that the *anterior* tibials are supplied by the *deep* peroneal nerve.

Biomechanical research by Hunt *et al.* (2001) suggests that peroneus longus has an important role to play in causing eversion after heel contact in the gait cycle. It acts to stabilise the forefoot after heel rise, whereas peroneus brevis seems to have a role in preventing lateral rotation of the leg over the foot later on in the stance phase of gait.

What do the retinaculae do?

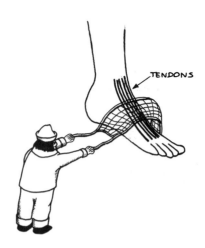

TENDONS

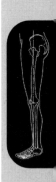

Muscles acting on the toes

Complete this table

Muscle	Action	Origin	Insertion	Nerve supply
Extensor hallucis longus				
Extensor digitorum longus				
Flexor hallucis longus This is important during the push off phase of walking				
Flexor digitorum longus				

Muscles of the lower limb

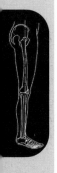

Intrinsic muscles of the foot (the four layers)

(Intrinsic muscles, i.e. they have origin and insertion within the foot.)

Complete this table

Muscle	Action	Origin	Insertion	Nerve supply
Superficial layer Abductor hallucis Flexor digitorum brevis Abductor digiti minimi				
Middle layer Tendon of flexor hallucis longus (fhl) Tendon of flexor digitorum longus (fdl) Flexor digitorum accessorius Lumbricals				
Deep layer Flexor hallucis brevis Adductor hallucis brevis				
Interosseous layer Plantar interossei Dorsal interossei	Revision aids: remember the words DAB & PAD. *Dorsal Abduct DAB Plantar Adduct PAD* (note – same applies in the hand)			

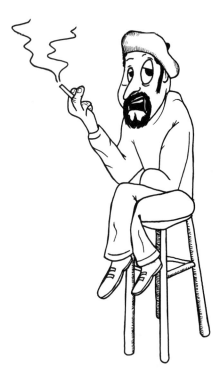

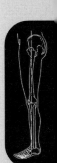

Medial plantar nerve supplies,
Abductor Hall 'neath which it lies,
Flexors brevis, dig and Hall
And the first lumbrical.

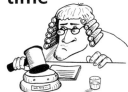

Judgement time

It is now time for you to assess whether or not you have achieved the learning outcomes at the start of this chapter.

You need to be able to tick each of these boxes, if you cannot, return to the relevant section of the chapter.

Can you now describe in writing and verbally the:

❑ Origin
❑ Insertion
❑ Action
❑ Functional (applied) anatomy
❑ Nerve supply

of the muscles contained in this chapter?

CHAPTER 4

NERVES OF THE LOWER LIMB

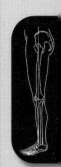

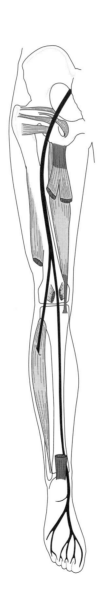

Nerves of the lower limb

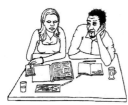
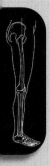

THE SACRAL PLEXUS

The term 'plexus' refers to a network of nerves or blood vessels. The nervous system features a number of these networks, where autonomic and voluntary nerve fibres join together. These networks include the brachial plexus (shoulder), the cervical plexus (neck), the coccygeal plexus (coccyx), and sacral or lumbosacral plexus (lower back).

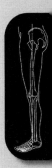

The lumbar plexus.

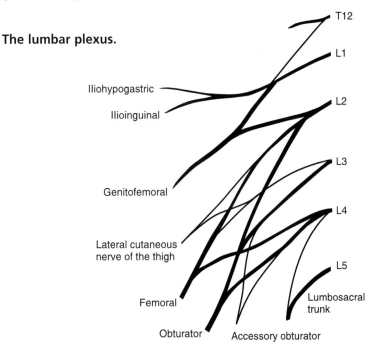

The sacral plexus.

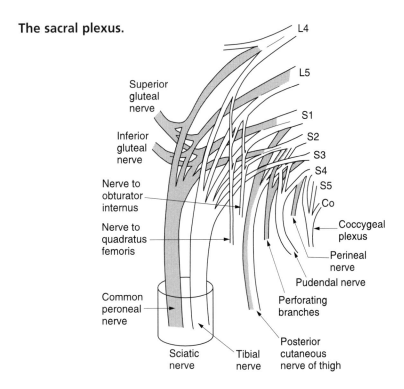

THE SCIATIC NERVE

The sciatic nerve (largest in the body) branches off the spinal cord between the fourth lumbar and third sacral vertebrae (L4, 5, S1, 2, 3). It extends down the centre of the posterior of the thigh. It appears as one single nerve until it reaches the apex of the popliteal fossa when it splits into two, the common peroneal and tibial nerves (remember though that strictly speaking it has always been two distinct nerves from the gluteal region). It innervates the hamstrings. Inflammation of the sciatic nerve, a condition known as sciatica, is a common problem and gives rise to referred pain (pain felt in a place other than where the actual problem is). At the apex of the popliteal fossa, it divides into the tibial and common peroneal nerves.

The tibial nerve branches off of the sciatic nerve and distally, divides into anterior and posterior branches. These branches innervate the muscles of the lower leg, ankle, and foot.

The peroneal nerves include the common, superficial, and deep peroneal nerves. Originating in the sciatic nerves, which branch off

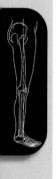

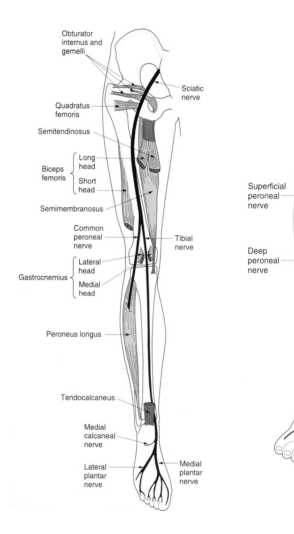

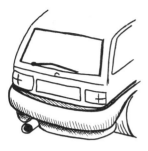

the spinal cord between the fourth lumbar and third sacral vertebrae, these nerves extend to the calf muscles, the skin of the top of the foot, and the toes.

The common peroneal nerve can often be palpated as it winds around the neck of the fibula; it may be compressed by a plaster cast which is too tight, and this may cause a foot drop – why?

Also, it is at exactly the same height as the bumper on a car – so it is quite vulnerable to being damaged.

THE FEMORAL NERVE

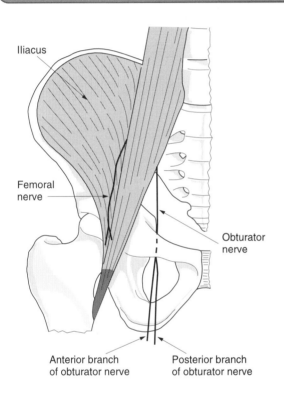

Iliacus

Femoral nerve

Obturator nerve

Anterior branch of obturator nerve

Posterior branch of obturator nerve

The femoral nerve branches off of the spinal cord between the second and fourth lumbar vertebrae (L2, 3, 4). It extends down the anterior of the thigh to supply the muscles and skin of the leg, including the thigh, knee, part of the calf, the ankle and the foot.

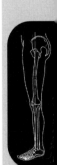

DERMATOMES

A dermatome is the area of skin supplied by a particular nerve root level. Note that there are differences from one textbook to the next, and from one human to the next.

So what? Well, it is possible for two people to have damage to the same nerve root level, but to have different symptoms. Dermatomes are important as they can act as strong clues when you are attempting to make a diagnosis. Speaking from personal experience, I hurt my back several years ago and it resulted in sciatic pain, and pins and needles (paraesthesia) down the inside of my shin, including my big toe. I am confident that my problem occurred at L4 level. You also need to know the myotomes of the body (the same as above but this term relates to muscles supplied by a particular nerve root level). For example the quadriceps is supplied by L2, 3, 4 and 'C3, 4 and 5 keep the diaphragm alive'.

Lower limb dermatomes.

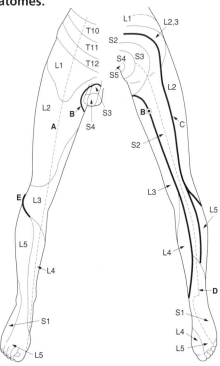

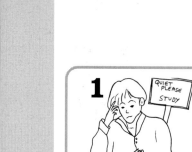

1 **Make sure that you understand the following:**

1 Structure of a mixed spinal nerve

2 Function of a mixed spinal nerve

3 Dermatomes

4 Myotomes.

Complete a summary of the:

1 Functional

2 Motor

3 Sensory loss.

That would occur in the following scenarios:

1 A patient has their common peroneal nerve severed by a traffic accident at the level of the neck of the fibula.

2 A patient is stabbed in the popliteal fossa, completely severing the tibial nerve.

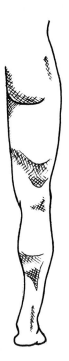

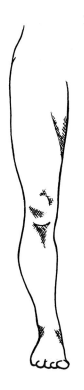

On these legs, draw the:

☞ sciatic
☞ obturator
☞ femoral nerves.

Now, draw the dermatomes of the lower limb on these legs.

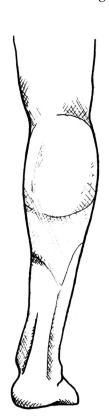

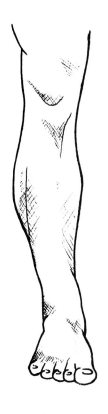

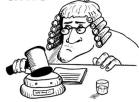

Judgement time

Can you describe (written and orally):

❑ root level
❑ relations
❑ major branches
❑ innervations
❑ signs and symptoms resulting from lesions of these nerves?
    ❑ sacral and lumbar plexuses

❑ sciatic nerve
❑ common peroneal nerve
❑ superficial peroneal nerve
❑ deep peroneal nerve
❑ tibial nerve
❑ medial/lateral plantar nerves.

❑ Do you know the gross structure, root level and location of the obturator and femoral nerves?
❑ Do you know the dermatomes of the lower limb?

135

CHAPTER
5

BONES OF THE UPPER LIMB

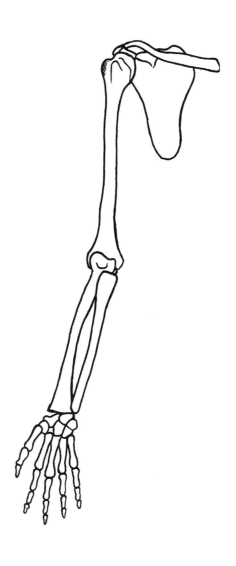

Bones of the upper limb

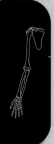

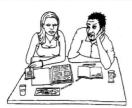

LEARNING OUTCOMES

Upon completion of this chapter and the relevant theory/practical sessions you should be able to:

1 Describe in detail the structure and function of all of the bones of the upper limb.

2 Be able to palpate these bony points (on two models of different gender).

❑ Spine of scapula

❑ Inferior angle of scapula

❑ Acromion process

❑ Acromioclavicular joint

❑ Sternoclavicular joint

❑ Coracoid process

❑ Clavicle

❑ Greater tuberosity of humerus

❑ Medial and lateral epicondyles of humerus

❑ Olecranon

❑ Radial head

❑ Ulnar styloid

❑ Radial styloid

❑ Pisiform

❑ Hook of hamate

❑ Metacarpals

❑ Phalanges.

3 Be able to identify the bony attachments/origin and insertion of the muscles and ligaments listed in Chapters 6 and 7.

THE BARE BONES

The scapula

The scapula (shoulder blade) is a roughly triangular shape; with the clavicle or collar bone it forms the pectoral or shoulder girdle. The scapula has two thick borders, yet if you hold one up to a bright light, the centre is so thin that it is translucent (allows light through).

PROFESSOR ASKS

Why is the central portion of the scapula so thin?

Clue: what attaches to the medial and lateral borders of the scapula?

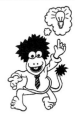

The humerus articulates with the scapula to form the shoulder or glenohumeral joint. This articulation takes place at the glenoid cavity, located at the upper, lateral angle of the scapula. The articular surface of the glenoid is about one-third the size of the articular surface of the humeral head. This is important to know because it means that from the bone point of view the shoulder joint is inherently unstable.

The posterior of the scapula features a laterally running line, which separates the surface into two unequally sized parts. This spine continues laterally and projects into the coracoid and the acromion (the acromion articulates with the lateral end of the clavicle). Both of these projections serve as anchors for muscle and connective tissue attachments; the spine and the acromion house the powerful trapezius and deltoid muscles. The shoulder joint and girdle are very mobile, but at the expense of some stability (it is much easier to dislocate a shoulder than a hip).

The shoulder joint may be considered as a mobile joint on a mobile platform, whereas the hip joint is basically a mobile joint on a fixed platform (the pelvis).

Many conditions and pathologies affect the shoulder: fractures, tendon and muscle problems, bursitis, etc. You need to fully understand the anatomy, function and biomechanics of the shoulder well in order to effectively diagnose and treat patients.

Off we go (again!).

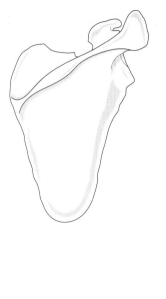

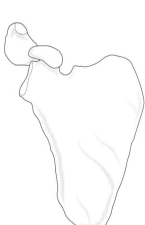

Add these labels:

- ☞ supraspinous fossa
- ☞ infraspinous fossa
- ☞ acromion
- ☞ suprascapular notch
- ☞ inferior angle
- ☞ medial border
- ☞ lateral border
- ☞ coracoid process
- ☞ glenoid fossa.

Hold a scapula in your hand. Position it so that you are looking directly at the glenoid fossa (i.e. sideways on, as shown below).

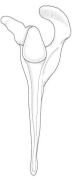

Could you label the following?

- ☞ coracoid process
- ☞ acromion
- ☞ infraglenoid tubercle
- ☞ supraglenoid tubercle

- ☞ lateral border
- ☞ inferior angle
- ☞ glenoid fossa.

PROFESSOR ASKS

- ☞ Which bones have an articulation with the scapula?
- ☞ How is the stability of the scapula maintained?
- ☞ What does supraspinous mean?
- ☞ What does infraglenoid mean?

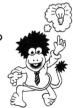

PROFESSOR SAYS

Make sure that you can describe the scapula and clavicle to another person, and articulate them together.

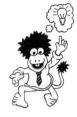

Answers
- ☞ The clavicle and the humerus
- ☞ By soft tissues – muscles in particular
- ☞ Above the spine
- ☞ Below the glenoid.

BODY POINTS – THE SHOULDER

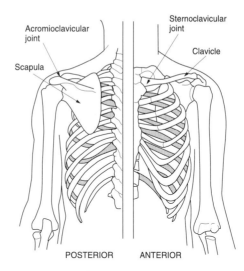

☞ Hold a scapula – describe it to your partner (partner – time how long it is before they run out of words).

☞ Hold a humerus – describe it to your partner (partner – time how long it is before they run out of words).

☞ Find and draw on your model:

❏ Spine of scapula
❏ Acromion
❏ Coracoid
❏ Greater tuberosity
❏ Humerus
❏ Sternum
❏ Xiphoid
❏ Medial border scapula
❏ Inferior angle scapula
❏ Medial and lateral humeral epicondyles.

THE CLAVICLE

The clavicle or collar bone is a long, slightly curving bone which forms the anterior part of each shoulder girdle. Located above the first rib on each side, each clavicle attaches to the sternum medially and laterally. The clavicle joins with the acromion process to form the acromioclavicular joint (ACJ). The clavicle acts to brace the scapula and gives the shoulder girdle mobility and stability. It houses some important ligaments and is important in controlling the way in which the shoulder girdle moves (scapulohumeral rhythm).

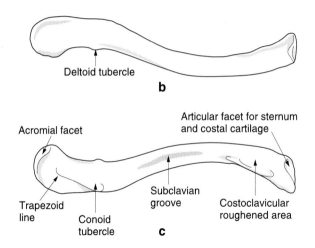

Deltoid tubercle

b

Acromial facet

Articular facet for sternum
and costal cartilage

Trapezoid
line

Conoid
tubercle

Subclavian
groove

Costoclavicular
roughened area

c

THE HUMERUS

The humerus is the long bone of the upper arm. Its head is articulated with the scapula at the shoulder joint and its distal end articulates with the radius and ulna, forming the elbow joint.

The humerus

Add labels.

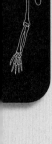

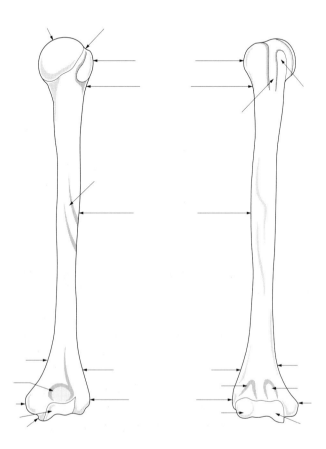

Labels

1	7
2	8
3	9
4	10
5	11
6	12

PROFESSOR ASKS

☞ Which joint is at the proximal end of the humerus?
☞ Which joints are at the distal end of the humerus?
☞ In what ways are the humerus and the femur alike?
☞ In what ways are the humerus and the femur different?

THE RADIUS

The radius is one of the two long arm bones (the other is the ulna) that form the forearm. The radius articulates at each end with the ends of the ulna, with the humerus at the elbow, and some of the carpal bones at the wrist. When the hand is turned with the palm facing up (supination) the radius is on the lateral side. When the hand is placed with the palm down (pronated) the radius crosses over the ulna in mid forearm.

Bones of the upper limb

THE ULNA

The ulna articulates at each end with the radius and with the humerus at the elbow. The ulna is always on the medial (little finger) side of the forearm.

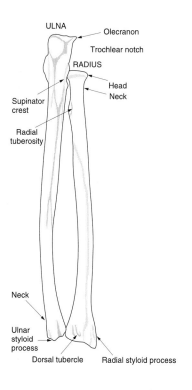

How do I remember which bone articulates with which part of the humerus?

The radius is so **radiant** that the humerus just **capitulates** and gives in (**radius = capitulum**).

The ulna is **un**believably stubborn and **tri**vial (**ul**na = **tro**chlea).

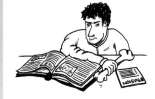

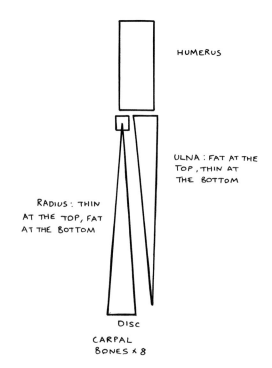

THE HAND

Each hand is made up of 27 bones. Eight of these bones form the compact arrangement of the wrist or carpus. These carpal bones include two rows of four bones (see diagrams). The distal row articulates with the five metacarpals and the proximal bones articulate with the wrist joint. The long metacarpals form the broad structure of the hand and they in turn articulate with the phalanges.

The bones of the fingers are called phalanges (singular = phalanx) – the same as in the foot. Each finger has three phalanges, with the exception of the thumb, which has two. The end of each phalanx is bulbous at the site of articulation with other bones.

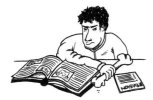

How do I remember the eight bones of the carpus?

SIMPLY (scaphoid)	**L**EARN (lunate)	**T**HE (triquetral)	**P**ARTS (pisiform)
THAT (trapezium)	**T**HE (trapezoid)	**C**ARPUS (capitate)	**H**AS (hamate)

Another rhyme to remember the carpal bones!

Some	Lovers	Try	Positions
That	They	Can't	Handle

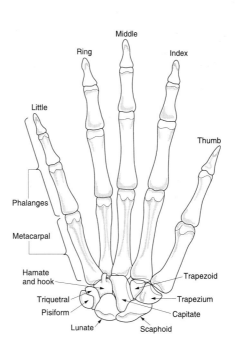

Your notes on the carpal bones.

Scaphoid
Lunate
Triquetral
Pisiform
Trapezium
Trapezoid
Capitate
Hamate

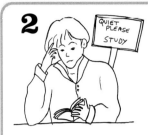

The metacarpals.

- Draw them
- Make notes on each
- Classify the bones
- Identify their palpable landmarks on a model.

The proximal phalanges.

- Draw them
- Make notes on each
- Classify the bones
- Identify their palpable landmarks on a model.

The intermediate phalanges.

- Draw them
- Make notes on each
- Classify the bones
- Identify their palpable landmarks on a model.

The distal phalanges.
- Draw them
- Make notes on each
- Classify the bones
- Identify their palpable landmarks on a model.

Look up the sesamoid bones in the hand.

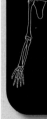

Bones of the upper limb

Judgement time

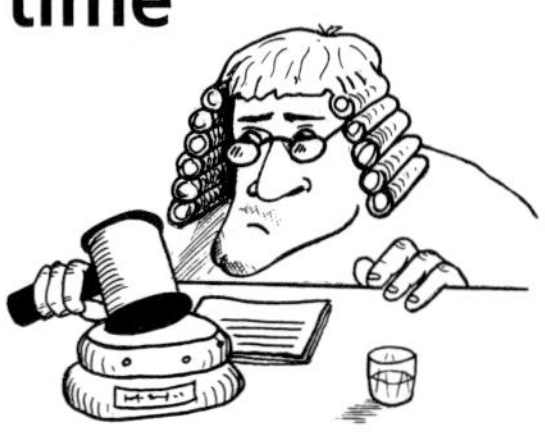

Theory

You need to be able to describe and identify all the features of bones included in this chapter.

Practical - bony points and landmarks

You must be able to find on a model the following:

❑ Clavicle (whole length)

❑ Acromion

❑ Coracoid process

❑ Head of humerus

❑ Radial styloid

❑ Ulnar styloid

❑ Posterior border of ulna

❑ Sternal notch

❑ Spine of scapula

❑ Inferior angle scapula

❑ Greater tuberosity humerus

❑ Medial epicondyle humerus

❑ Lateral epicondyle humerus

❑ Radial head

❑ Olecranon

❑ Head of ulna

❑ Metacarpals 1–5

❑ All proximal phalanges

❑ All terminal phalanges

❑ Pisiform

❑ Scaphoid

❑ Hook of hamate.

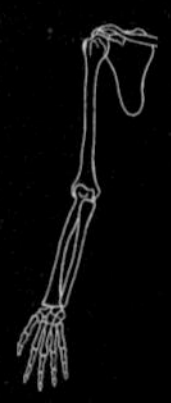

JOINTS OF THE UPPER LIMB

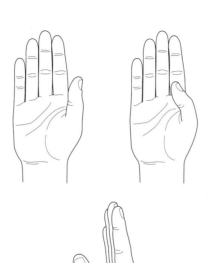

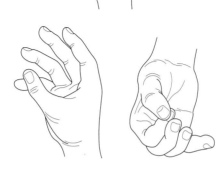

Joints of the upper limb

LEARNING OUTCOMES

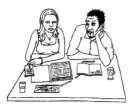

Upon completion of this chapter, the relevant lectures and practical sessions you should be able to:

1 Describe (for your written paper and orally for your exams) the structure of all joints of the upper limb including articular surfaces, movements possible, ligaments, capsule and other important features particular to that joint.

2 Describe (for your written paper and orally for your exams) the function of all joints of the upper limb.

3 Be able to relate 1 (above) to 2 (above).

4 Have a working knowledge of limiting factors to movements of the joints of the upper limb.

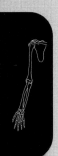

THE SHOULDER GIRDLE COMPLEX

THE JOINTS INVOLVED

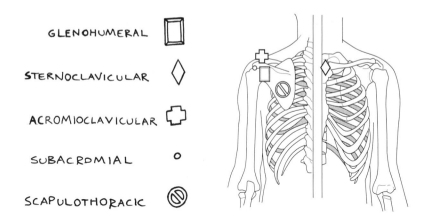

GLENOHUMERAL

STERNOCLAVICULAR

ACROMIOCLAVICULAR

SUBACROMIAL

SCAPULOTHORACIC

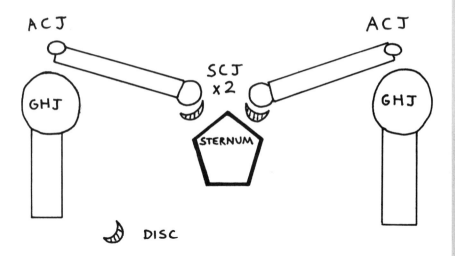

ACJ   ACJ

GHJ   SCJ x2   GHJ

STERNUM

DISC

The *plane* of the scapula

As the wings of a *plane* sweep at an angle, so does the scapula as it sits on the thorax.

Movements at the hip were described in pure anatomical planes. Well, just to make your student life a little more difficult this is not the case for the shoulder joint.

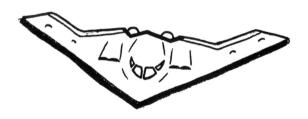

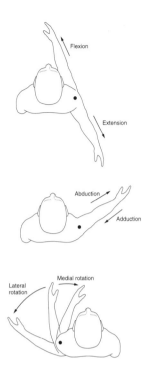

More on the plane of the scapula

Think back to what you learned about the hip joint. Remember how flexion was in the frontal plane, abduction was in a transverse plane and so on – the situation at the shoulder is not that simple. If you look at a person's scapulae, you will see that they lie posteriorly and also slightly protracted in the resting position. For this reason measurements of the shoulder joint are off-set slightly.

- There is a joint between the humerus and the scapula called....
- There is a joint between sternum and clavicle called.................
- There is a joint between acromion and clavicle called................
- What is the subacromial joint? ....
- What is the scapulothoracic joint?...

Answers

- The glenohumeral joint
- The sternoclavicular joint
- The acromioclavicular joint
- The false joint formed underneath the acromion and including the subacromial bursa
- The term for the site where the scapula 'floats' on the thoracic wall.

The sterno-clavicular joint (SCJ)

Believe it or not, this is the only bony point of contact between the arm and the chest. Remember it by comparing it to the shoulder protectors worn by American soccer players which have a fastener over the SCJ – with thanks to James Baldwin.

The sterno-clavicular joint.

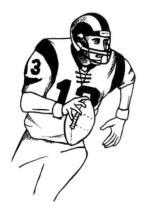

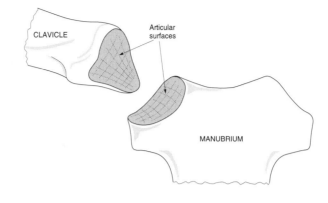

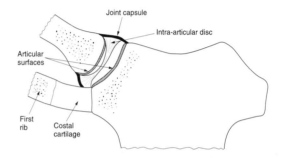

It is between the medial end of the clavicle and the superolateral angle of the sternum and 1st costal cartilage. The joint surfaces are not congruent – but this is minimised by the presence of an intra-articular disc.

<table>
<tr><td>

The fibrous capsule of the SCJ

</td><td>

This is in the form of a sleeve around the joint. It is strong and is reinforced by anterior and posterior sternoclavicular ligaments and an interclavicular ligament.

</td></tr>
</table>

Label the diagram below

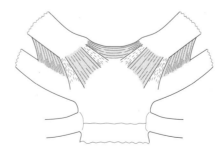

☞ The anterior sternoclavicular ligament
☞ The posterior sternoclavicular ligament
☞ The interclavicular ligament
☞ The intra-articular disc.

The SCJ is divided into two distinct cavities by the presence of a disc. The joint therefore has two synovial membranes! The disc:

☞ Improves joint congruency. What does this statement mean?
☞ Cushions the joint
☞ Acts as a ligament.

(Holding down the medial end of the clavicle against the sternum.)

Movements of the sternoclavicular joint

There are five degrees of freedom of motion:

❏ elevation
❏ depression
❏ protraction
❏ retraction
❏ axial rotation.

The axis for all these except axial rotation is the costoclavicular ligament.

Movements of the clavicle

Think of the clavicle as a see-saw, with the pivot being the costoclavicular ligament (cc below); as one end goes up, the other falls.

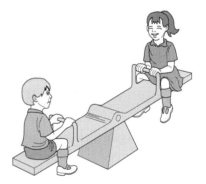

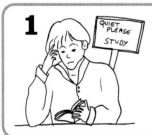

1 **Make a more detailed study of the costoclavicular ligament, including clavicular movements and limiting factors to movements.**

The acromioclavicular joint (ACJ)

This joint is synovial between the flat facet on the lateral end of the clavicle and the flat facet on the anteromedial border of the acromion. Both surfaces are covered in fibrocartilage. Because of the shape and alignments of the surfaces, dislocations of the ACJ usually result in the acromion being displaced downwards and underneath the clavicle. The capsule is thickest above (superiorly) and is reinforced by trapezius. It is lined by synovial membrane. It usually possesses a wedge-shaped disc which increases joint congruency.

No muscles move the ACJ alone, none connect the two bones, but all movements of the scapula include movements of both (ACJ and SCJ).

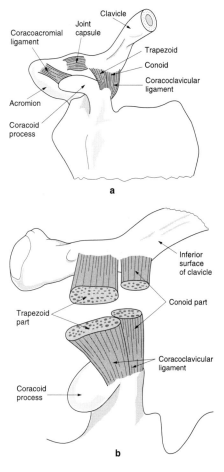

(2 distinct parts.)

The coracoclavicular ligament

Conoid part	Trapezoid part
Attachments	Attachments
Structure	Structure
Function (limits forwards movement of the scapula)	Function (limits backwards movement of the scapula)

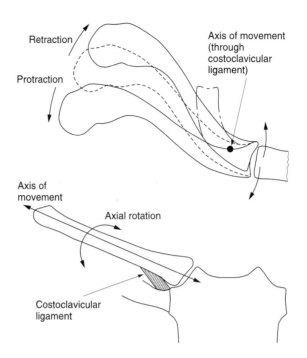

Retraction

Protraction

Axis of movement
(through
costoclavicular
ligament)

Axis of
movement

Axial rotation

Costoclavicular
ligament

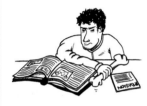

Remember the two parts of the coracoclavicular ligament (cc lig): Cutting corn requires a Con Traption (coracoid and trapezoid).

SCAPULAR ROTATION

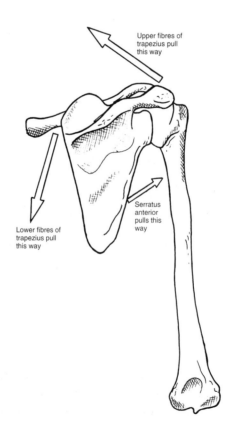

Upper fibres of
trapezius pull
this way

Serratus
anterior
pulls this
way

Lower fibres of
trapezius pull
this way

The glenohumeral joint

If you thought of the hip as an egg in an egg cup, think of the shoulder joint as a football resting on a saucer; the ball (humeral head) is too big for the saucer (glenoid) and the saucer is not really deep enough to stabilise the football.

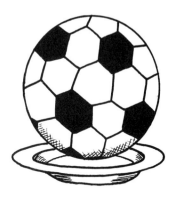

So if the shoulder had to rely on the shape of its bones alone it would be very unstable. It needs help. It overcomes this problem by relying heavily on soft tissues which act as dynamic ligaments (the rotator cuff) rather like guy ropes on a tent.

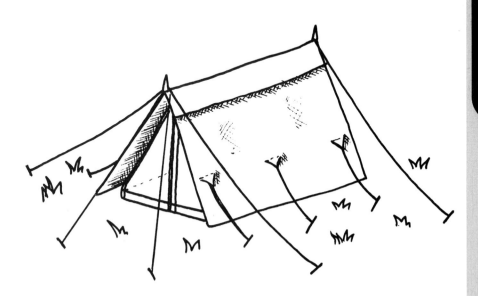

What does the shoulder joint do?

The function of the human shoulder is to place the hand in a functional position; hence it needs to be a very mobile joint but still keep a large amount of stability, fine movements, co-ordination, etc.

Joints of the upper limb

Is the shoulder joint working in each of these activities?

If you answered *yes*, what is the shoulder doing for each?

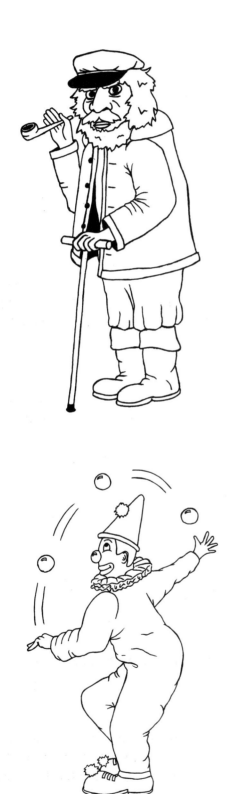

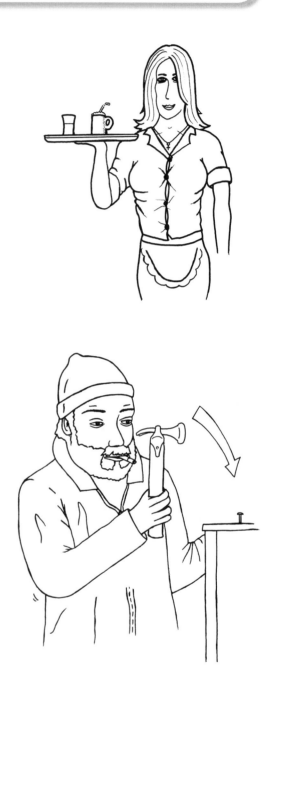

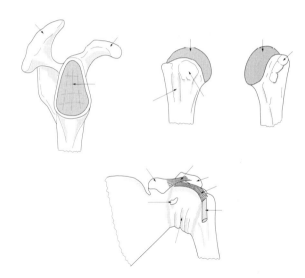

Add labels to the above diagrams.

Stop press: it *was* thought that the rotator cuff was the single most important factor in maintaining shoulder joint stability – it is now thought that also the negative pressure within the capsule helps cohesion of the bony surfaces. The biceps muscle also plays a role (see Chapter 7).

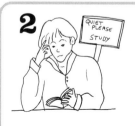

☞ Make sure that you fully understand the joints, bones and ligaments of the shoulder girdle.

☞ Can you discuss how these joints function in a living body?

☞ Why does the arrangement in the shoulder need to be different to that in the hip?

☞ Could you point out the structures of the shoulder girdle on
 ❑ A model?
 ❑ A skeleton?

☞ Would you be able to talk about the shoulder girdle to:
 ❑ An examiner in your practical exams?
 ❑ A patient with *no* knowledge of anatomy?
 ❑ An orthopaedic surgeon?

☞ How would you modify your answers for each case above?

Stop press: the glenohumeral joint possesses a labrum rather like that found in the hip joint. It is increasingly being thought that problems with the labrum may be responsible for shoulder pain and instability (Jobe 1996).

Joints of the upper limb

SCAPULOHUMERAL RHYTHM OR IS IT HUMEROSCAPULAR RHYTHM?

Abduction/elevation of the human shoulder girdle is complex. Make a more detailed study of this – it is very important that you understand this. Below is a simplified account of how it happens.

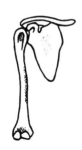

Starting point – arm by side.

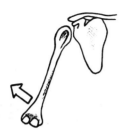

Look up the latest biomechanical explanation for which muscles are active during this part of abduction.

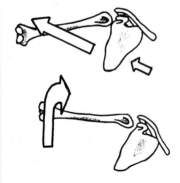

Into more abduction, the scapula starts to rotate and tries to 'Catch up' but never quite makes it. Force couple in action. Which muscles though? The greatest amount of relative scapular movement according to Bagg & Forrest (1988) is between 80 and 140° of arm abduction.

At approximately 90° of abduction, conjunct rotation of humerus has to happen to prevent the greater tuberosity of the humerus hitting the underside of the acromion.

The final few degrees of elevation is not by shoulder joint at all – it is done by scapular protraction=serratus anterior. If serratus anterior were weak what would you detect on examination?

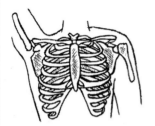

TEST YOURSELF

Which muscles are represented by the three arrows on the scapula below?

So what – why do I need to know?

Which muscles do these arrows represent on this scapula?

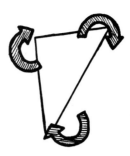

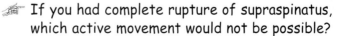
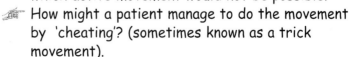

Answers
- Upper fibres trapezius
- Lower fibres of trapezius
- Serratus anterior.

SO WHAT – WHY DO I NEED TO KNOW?

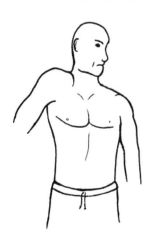

You need to understand a normal humeroscapular rhythm before you can spot an abnormal one – if a patient has rheumatoid arthritis of the shoulder for example, the rotator cuff becomes severely degenerated and cannot perform its task of initiating abduction and stabilising the humeral head. The head of the humerus 'crashes' upwards into the underside of the acromion. Deltoid is left to cope and the patient will instead elevate the shoulder girdle first rather than as shown above. This makes the patient appear to hunch the shoulder – this is another important reason for you to expose the area when examining movements – it might appear that the man in the picture had 70° of abduction – he actually only has 20° at the glenohumeral joint!

PROFESSOR ASKS

- If you had complete rupture of supraspinatus, which active movement would not be possible?
- How might a patient manage to do the movement by 'cheating'? (sometimes known as a trick movement).
- Why do patients sometimes develop a painful shoulder on the affected side following a CVA (cerebrovascular accident or stroke)?

Answers

☞ Initiation of abduction.
☞ They might lift the arm with the other arm or use a swinging movement to overcome the first few degrees of abduction.
☞ Poor handling by people that overstretches soft tissues that have already lost tone and can result in instability and pain.

A STICKY PROBLEM

The capsule of the shoulder joint.

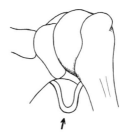

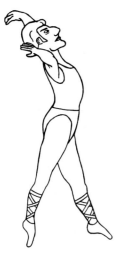

Look at how lax the glenohumeral capsule is inferiorly. This allows a huge range of movement at a normal glenohumeral joint.

These loose folds occasionally stick together, together with capsular contraction, severely restricting movements at the shoulder joint; this is a frozen shoulder – the correct term is adhesive capsulitis. A patient with this condition loses set proportions of movements – a capsular pattern.

You need to know the capsular patterns for the joints of the body.

HIP VERSUS SHOULDER JOINT

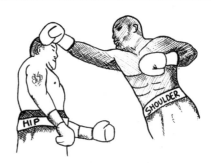

It might be useful for you to compare and contrast these two joints so that you can prove to yourself that your knowledge is increasing – or maybe not!

Complete this table

	Hip joint	Shoulder joint
Type of joint		
Degrees of freedom of movement		
Internal ligament		
Labrum		
Factors providing stability		
Factors allowing mobility		
Ease of dislocation		
Common direction of dislocation		
Major muscle groups		

GIVING YOU 'THE ELBOW' ⇐ A JOKE

PROFESSOR'S TIP

A fracture is the same as a break in medicine!

The elbow is an important joint as once again its function is to place the hand in a useful position – ask anybody who has a fractured elbow how difficult it is to wash and eat!

Joints of the upper limb

THE BONES OF THE ELBOW JOINT

🖐 Distal humerus
🖐 Proximal radius
🖐 Proximal ulna.

The distal humerus has a trochlea and a capitulum.

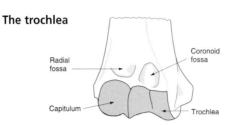

The trochlea

Radial fossa
Coronoid fossa
Capitulum
Trochlea

The capitulum

Olecranon fossa
Trochlea

Articulates with the ulna.　　　　Articulates with the radial head.

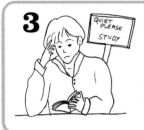

3

Using your classmates or friends, look at three male elbow joints and three female elbow joints.

Do they differ? How do they differ? Why do they differ?

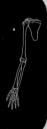

Label the elbow joint

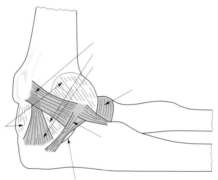

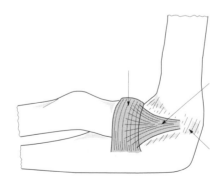

The elbow has strong collateral ligaments – bunched at the sides of the joint so as not to interfere with the movements of flexion and extension. Look at an elbow from the side, the trochlea notch bulges anteriorly at an angle of 45°; this allows more flexion to occur. The ulna deviates 10–15° in males and 20–25° in females.

The elbow joint capsule

A capsule envelops the joint, from the medial epicondyle to the coronoid/radial fossae, posteriorly it follows the capitulum and arches upwards around the olecranon.

The collateral ligaments

These are strong triangular bands blended with the capsule. They limit ab- and adduction. They are called the radial collateral and the ulnar collateral ligaments.

Palpation

Anteriorly muscles are in the way and the joint is not palpable. The joint line, however, is a line joining the two points, 1 cm below the lateral epicondyle and 2 cm below the medial epicondyle.

Stability

Stability comes from the elbow joint's bony shape; it is most stable in 90° of flexion (this is where most daily activities occur).

Movement

Movement of the elbow consists of flexion and extension, occurring through the carrying angle. Accessory movements of ab- and adduction are possible with the elbow in extension.

There is also a joint between the radius and ulna (superior radio-ulnar joint) and the radius and ulna also articulate with one another inferiorly (no prizes for guessing the name of this joint!).

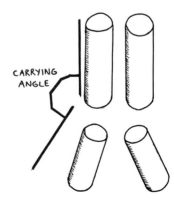

MALE ELBOW

FEMALE ELBOW

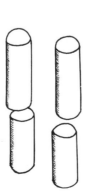

CARRYING ANGLE

RADIO-ULNAR MOVEMENTS

Humero-ulnar joint	Radio-ulnar joint
Flexion	Pronation
Extension	Supination

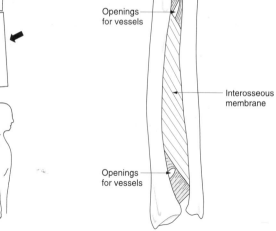

Limiting factors in the normal elbow

Flexion : soft tissue approximation.

Extension: bony block.

The radius and ulna articulated together.

BICEPS GETS IN THE WAY

BONY CONTACT KNOWN AS "END FEEL"

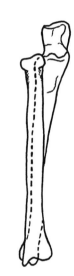

Oblique cord

Openings for vessels

Interosseous membrane

Openings for vessels

How to remember pronation and supination.

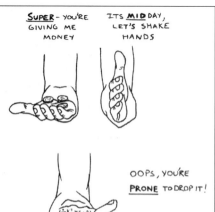

SUPER - YOU'RE GIVING ME MONEY

ITS **MID** DAY, LET'S SHAKE HANDS

OOPS, YOU'RE **PRONE** TO DROP IT!

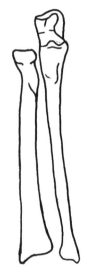

The annular ligament grips the radial head like the cuff on a crutch.

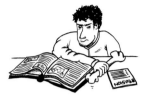

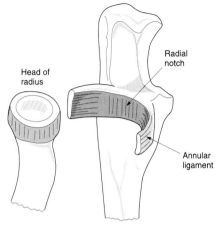

Head of radius

Radial notch

Annular ligament

THE ANNULAR LIGAMENT GRIPS THE RADIAL HEAD LIKE THE CUFF ON A CRUTCH

THE WRIST JOINT

RADIUS AND ULNA

The wrist is a complex joint and its function is closely linked with hand and radio-ulnar joint function. The wrist joint possesses an intra-articular disc. Arthroscopy of the wrist is now common and repairs to the disc complex can be performed using keyhole techniques (Cober & Trumble 2001).

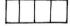 **Carpal bones.**

Transverse section through the wrist.

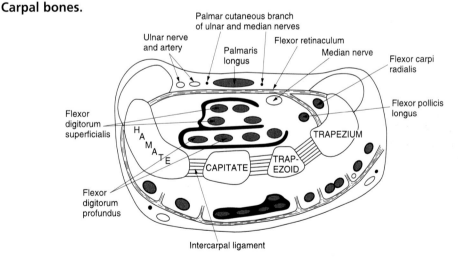

Palmar cutaneous branch of ulnar and median nerves

Ulnar nerve and artery

Palmaris longus

Flexor retinaculum

Median nerve

Flexor carpi radialis

Flexor pollicis longus

Flexor digitorum superficialis

HAMATE

TRAPEZIUM

CAPITATE

TRAP-EZOID

Flexor digitorum profundus

Intercarpal ligament

The wrist possesses collateral ligaments and movements possible include flexion extension, abduction and adduction.

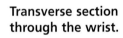 Two rows of four bones
Minimal movement between bones
Dorsal, palmar, interosseous intercarpal ligaments present.

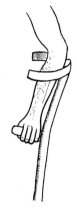

The carpus.

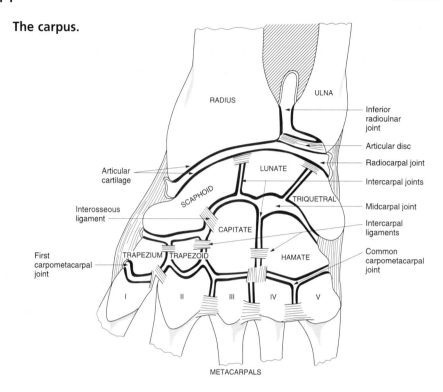

| Midcarpal joint | 🖎 Between the two rows of carpal bones
🖎 Possesses dorsal, palmar, interosseous ligaments and incorporates radial and ulnar collateral ligaments. |

| Midcarpal movements | 🖎 Flexion – 50° possible
🖎 Extension – 35° possible
🖎 Abduction – 8° possible
🖎 Adduction – 15° possible. |

| Intermetacarpal joints | 🖎 Plane synovial
🖎 Palmar and dorsal ligaments
🖎 Small amplitude gliding movements occur here. |

| Carpometacarpal joint of the thumb | 🖎 Mobile but stable too (remember the hip joint?)
🖎 Between trapezium and base of 1st metacarpal
🖎 The classic example of a saddle joint. |

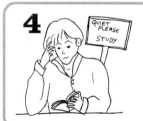

4 **Summarise the movements and limiting factors to movements of these joints.**

Metacarpohalan-geal joints (MCP)

☞ Synovial condyloid joint
☞ Two degrees of freedom of movement: flexion/extension and abduction/adduction
☞ Some accessory rotation possible, in fact essential for normal movement, e.g. when gripping a ball.

Interphalangeal joints

On your own:

☞ Classify them.
☞ What are their main ligaments?
☞ Which movements are possible?

MOVEMENTS OF THE THUMB

Just to make life difficult for you the thumb does not lie in the same plane as the other fingers; as a result all measurements are different and can appear confusing at times. You need to understand the movement of the thumb, so I want you to add notes.

Complete this table

Movement	Definition	Muscles producing it	Functional example	Limiting factors
Thumb flexion				
Thumb extension				
Thumb adduction				
Thumb abduction				
Thumb opposition				

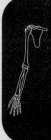

Joints of the upper limb

Complete the table for the upper limb

Joint	Limiting factors (in the normal joint)

Shoulder
 	
  Flexion
 	
  Extension
 	
  Abduction
 	
  Adduction
 	
  Internal rotation
 	
  External rotation
 	
  ACJ
 	
  SCJ	

Elbow
 	
  Flexion
 	
  Extension	

Superior radio-ulnar joint
 	
  Pronation
 	
  Supination	

Wrist joint
 	
  Flexion
 	
  Extension
 	
  Abduction
 	
  Adduction	

Metacarpophalangeal joints
 	
  Flexion
 	
  Extension
 	
  Abduction
 	
  Adduction	

Interphalangeal joints
 	
  Flexion
 	
  Extension	

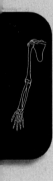

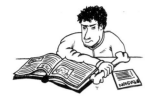

How can I remember what passes through the carpal tunnel?

The carpal tunnel is like the M25 on a bad day, a busy place and not much room for mistakes.

Think of

4 professors	= 4 <u>prof</u>undus tendons
On **4 s**cooters	= 4 <u>s</u>uperficialis tendons
Nearby is a **fairly polite lady**	= <u>FPL</u> tendon
with **m**oney	= <u>m</u>edian nerve.

Judgement time

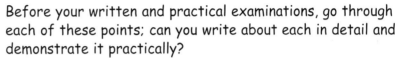

Before your written and practical examinations, go through each of these points; can you write about each in detail and demonstrate it practically?

You should be able to identify practically on a model and write about in detail for written exams:

Shoulder (glenohumeral)

❑ Joint line
❑ Movements
❑ Limiting factors to movement
❑ Bones involved
❑ Classification.

Acromio-clavicular and sternoclavicular

❑ Joint line
❑ Movements
❑ Limiting factors to movement
❑ Bones involved
❑ Classification
❑ Main ligaments.

Elbow joint

❑ Palpate location
❑ Joint line
❑ Classification
❑ Ligaments
❑ Limiting factors to movement.

Superior radio-ulnar joint

❑ Joint line
❑ Movements
❑ Limiting factors to movement
❑ Bones involved
❑ Classification.

- ❑ Three lateral ligaments
- ❑ Medial (deltoid) ligament.

Inferior radio-ulnar joint

- ❑ Movements
- ❑ Limiting factors to movement
- ❑ Bones involved
- ❑ Classification
- ❑ Ligaments.

Wrist joint

- ❑ Bones involved
- ❑ Classification
- ❑ Movements possible
- ❑ Main ligaments.

Midcarpal joint

- ❑ Bones involved
- ❑ Classification
- ❑ Movements possible
- ❑ Main ligaments.

Metacarpo-phalangeal and interphalangeal joints

- ❑ Bones involved
- ❑ Classification
- ❑ Movements possible
- ❑ Main ligaments.

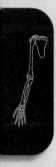

MUSCLES OF THE UPPER LIMB

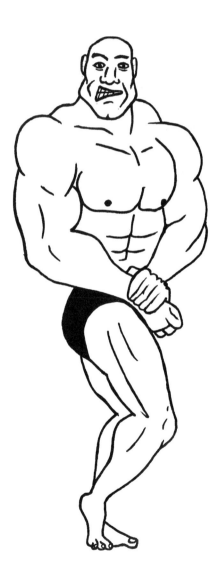

Muscles of the upper limb

LEARNING OUTCOMES

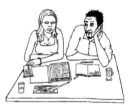

Upon completion of this chapter and the relevant lectures and practical sessions you should be able to describe in writing and verbally the:

1 Origin

2 Insertion

3 Action

4 Functional (applied) anatomy

5 Nerve supply

of the muscles contained in this chapter.

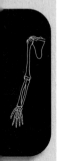

MUSCLES AROUND THE SHOULDER GIRDLE

The muscles of the shoulder girdle are of the following types.

- Elevators
- Depressors
- Protractors
- Retractors
- Lateral rotators
- Medial rotators.

Shoulder girdle elevators

Complete this table

Muscle	Action	Origin	Insertion	Nerve supply
Levator scapulae				
Upper fibres trapezius				

Shoulder girdle retractors

Complete this table

Muscle	Action	Origin	Insertion	Nerve supply
Rhomboid major				
Rhomboid minor				
Trapezius				

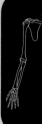

Shoulder girdle protractors

Complete this table

Muscle	Action	Origin	Insertion	Nerve supply
Serratus anterior				
Pectoralis minor				

Ask a model (topless!) to push against a wall with their elbows extended. Stand behind them and observe their scapulae. Serratus anterior works hard to prevent their nose hitting the wall – it is a similar movement to doing a 'press up'. If serratus anterior is weak, a 'winged scapula' results. This means that the scapula is not held against the thorax as it should be and 'sticks out' especially the medial border and inferior angle.

Serratus anterior.

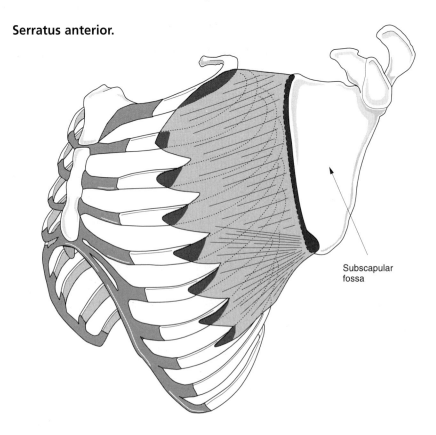

Subscapular fossa

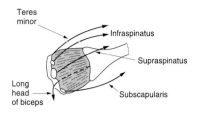

Teres minor — Infraspinatus — Supraspinatus — Long head of biceps — Subscapularis

The rotator cuff

Complete this table

Muscle	Action	Origin	Insertion	Nerve supply
Supraspinatus				
Subscapularis				
Infraspinatus				
Teres minor				

The rotator cuff is very important – you should know it in detail.

PROFESSOR ASKS

If the rotator cuff is so great, then why is there not a rotator cuff in the hip joint?

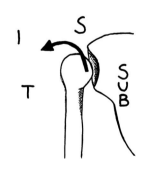

Answer

Doesn't need one – the hip is less reliant on soft tissues for its stability than the shoulder.

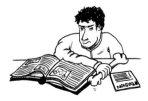

An easy way to remember their relative positions. *Remember*: SubSIT. Starting from the most anterior, this tells you their positions

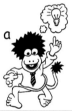

☞ **S** (ubscapularis)
☞ **S** (upraspinatus)
☞ **I** (nfraspinatus)
☞ **T** (eres minor).

Muscles of the upper limb

Supraspinatus

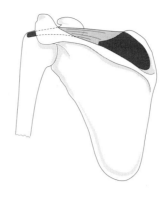

- What does 'supra' mean?
- What does 'spinatus' mean?
- Which other muscles make up the rotator cuff?
- What is the action of the rotator cuff?
- Supraspinatus lesions frequently exhibit a painful arc – what is this?

Answers

- Above
- The spine (of scapula)
- Infraspinatus teres minor subscapularis
- Acts as a set of dynamic ligaments controlling the position of the humeral head
- Pain felt in middle range abduction – consult a soft tissue injuries text.

More 'off the cuff' comments

One of the most important functions of the rotator cuff is to surround and support the humeral head. If I gave you a bundle of money (yeah right!) that you wanted to hold securely, you would grab it, wrapping your fingers around the money so that from all directions the money would be secure.

Think of the rotator cuff in this way, surrounding the head of the humerus to give the shoulder stability, yet adaptable enough to allow a large number of fine movements. A person who has suffered a stroke (cerebrovascular incident) may lose muscle tone in their rotator cuff – hence the shoulder becomes unstable and subluxes; it is quite common to find painful shoulders in these patients. Now you know why.

Stop press: one of the newer theories about how the shoulder joint maintains its stability focuses on the negative pressure within the joint – a bit like sucking the air out of a balloon, the edges of the balloon are held together. Bearing this in mind, why do some surgeons now believe that arthroscopy of the shoulder causes problems in itself?

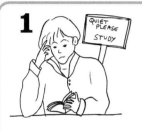

1 A friend comes to see you, he has been diagnosed as having a torn rotator cuff. Nobody has explained this to him and he is very worried about what this means exactly – write down what you would say to him. If you wish, show the finished product to a lecturer for their comments, better still, show it to a friend who knows nothing about anatomy – see if they understand it. It is one thing being able to write wonderful essays but no use to you if you cannot get the information across simply and in a form that is understood by non-health care professionals.

Deltoid

The deltoid muscle.

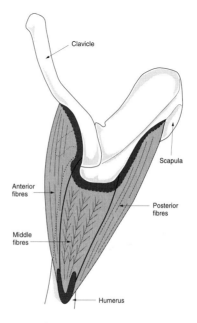

☞ The middle fibres of deltoid are multipennate, what does this statement mean?

☞ The anterior fibres of deltoid lie anterior to the glenohumeral joint therefore they will assist with .... of the shoulder

☞ The posterior fibres of deltoid lie posterior to the glenohumeral joint therefore they will assist with .... of the shoulder

☞ Which muscle assists deltoid by initiating abduction of the shoulder?

Answers

☞ Look it up in Chapter 1 under morphology of muscle
☞ Flexion
☞ Extension
☞ Supraspinatus.

Latissimus dorsi

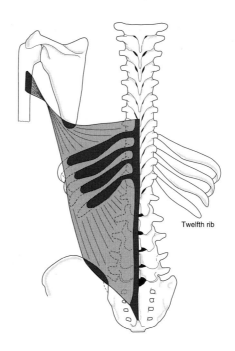

Twelfth rib

☞ This huge muscle gives bodybuilders their **V** shape.

☞ It has attachments as low as the ilium, so it can achieve hitching of the pelvis if its action is reversed (insertion remains fixed and origin moves instead). There is now research to suggest that the influence that this muscle has over the lumbosacral spine is minimal (Bogduk *et al*. 1998).

Trapezius

A = direction of pull of upper trapezius fibres
B = direction of pull of lower trapezius fibres
C = direction of pull of serratus anterior.

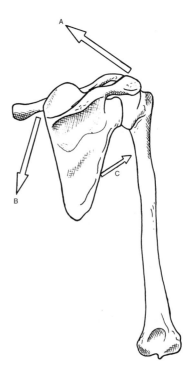

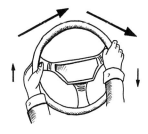

Combined force couple result is scapular rotation, rather like steering a car by using two opposite movements on either side of the wheel.

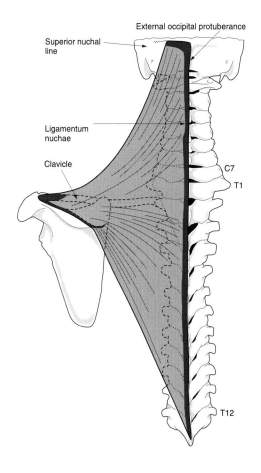

External occipital protuberance

Superior nuchal line

Ligamentum nuchae

Clavicle

C7

T1

T12

Shoulder flexors

Complete this table

Muscle	Action	Origin	Insertion	Nerve supply
Pectoralis major **(sternal head)** **(clavicular head)**				
Deltoid (anterior fibres)				
Biceps (long head)				
Coracobrachialis				

Muscles of the upper limb

Shoulder extensors

Complete this table

Muscle	Action	Origin	Insertion	Nerve supply
Latissimus dorsi				
Teres major				
Deltoid (posterior fibres)				
Triceps (long head)				

Shoulder adductors

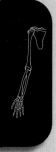

Complete this table

Muscle	Action	Origin	Insertion	Nerve supply
Coracobrachialis				
Pectoralis major				
Latissimus dorsi				
Teres major				

Complete this table

Muscle	Action	Origin	Insertion	Nerve supply
Subscapularis				
Teres major				
Latissimus dorsi				
Deltoid (anterior fibres)				
Pectoralis major 1. Sternal fibres 2. Clavicular fibres.				

Complete this table

Muscle	Action	Origin	Insertion	Nerve supply
Teres minor				
Infraspinatus				
Deltoid (posterior fibres)				

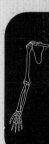

Muscles of the upper limb

Biceps brachii –
two heads are
better than one

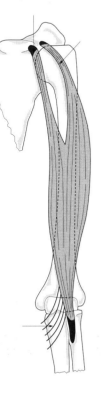

And the jokes just keep on coming!

On this diagram label the long and short heads and the bicipital aponeurosis of the biceps brachii.

- What does the word biceps mean?
- What does brachii mean?
- What does biceps do:

  (a) at the glenohumeral joint?
  (b) at the elbow joint?
  (c) at the radio-ulnar joint?
  (d) What signs and symptoms would you expect following a rupture (complete snapping) of the long head of biceps?

Andrews *et al.* (1985) made these observations about biceps:

'Only the biceps brachii traverses both the elbow joint and the shoulder joint. Additional forces are generated in the biceps tendon in its function as a shunt muscle to stabilise the glenohumeral joint during the throwing act.'

PROFESSOR SAYS

'Lets hear it for the left handers'

Supination is more powerful than pronation so left-handed people are better at removing screws that are stubborn!

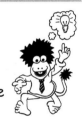

Answers

- Two heads
- Arm
- (a) Flexes the elbow joint; (b) flexion at the glenohumeral joint (via its long head); (c) supinates forearm
- Sudden snap may be felt. Shoulder pain (or not). Arm will take on appearance of Popeye muscle as muscle belly shunts distally.

PROFESSOR'S TIP

A symptom is what a person complains of, a sign is what can be measured or tested for.

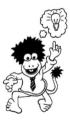

ELBOW FLEXORS

Complete this table

Muscle	Action	Origin	Insertion	Nerve supply
Biceps brachii				
Brachialis				
Brachioradialis				
Pronator teres				

TRICEPS

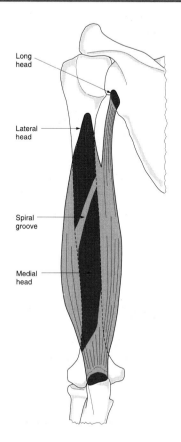

Long head

Lateral head

Spiral groove

Medial head

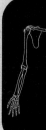

Muscles of the upper limb

Complete this table

Muscle	Action	Origin	Insertion	Nerve supply
Triceps				
Long head				
Lateral head				
Medial head				
Anconeus				

PRONATION AND SUPINATION

Complete this table

Muscle	Action	Origin	Insertion	Nerve supply
Pronator teres				
Pronator quadratus				
Biceps brachii				
Supinator				

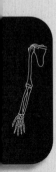

FLEXION AT THE WRIST JOINT

Complete this table

Muscle	Action	Origin	Insertion	Nerve supply
Flexor carpi ulnaris				
Flexor carpi radialis				
Flexor digitorum superficialis				
Flexor digitorum profundus				
Flexor pollicis longus				

Pollicis = thumb; hallux = toe.

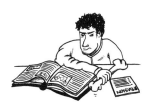

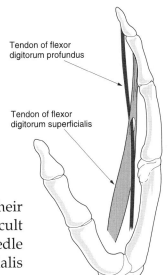

Tendon of flexor digitorum profundus

Tendon of flexor digitorum superficialis

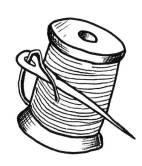

How to remember the tendons and their arrangement. It can be _profoundly_ difficult to thread unless you have a _super_ needle (_profundus_ threads through _super_ficialis tendon).

187

Muscles of the upper limb

EXTENSION AT THE WRIST JOINT

Complete this table

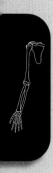

Muscle	Action	Origin	Insertion	Nerve supply
Extensor carpi radialis longus				
Extensor carpi radialis brevis				
Extensor carpi ulnaris				
Extensor digitorum				
Extensor indicis				
Extensor digiti minimi				
Extensor pollicis longus				
Extensor pollicis brevis				

FLEXION OF THE FINGERS/THUMB

Complete this table

Muscle	Action	Origin	Insertion	Nerve supply
Flexor digitorum superficialis				
Flexor digitorum profundus				
Lumbricals				
Flexor digiti minimi brevis				
Thumb Flexor pollicis longus				
Thumb Flexor pollicis brevis				

EXTENSION OF THE FINGERS/THUMB

Complete this table

Muscle	Action	Origin	Insertion	Nerve supply
Extensor digitorum				
Extensor digiti minimi				

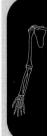

Muscles of the upper limb

Muscle	Action	Origin	Insertion	Nerve supply
Extensor indicis				
Interossei				
Lumbricals				
Thumb Extensor pollicis longus				
Thumb Extensor pollicis brevis				

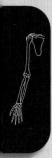

ABDUCTION/ADDUCTION/OPPOSITION OF THE THUMB

Complete this table

Muscle	Action	Origin	Insertion	Nerve supply
Abductor pollicis longus				
Abductor pollicis brevis				
Opponens pollicis				

Muscle	Action	Origin	Insertion	Nerve supply
Adductor pollicis				
Palmaris brevis				

ABDUCTION/ADDUCTION/OPPOSITION OF THE FINGERS

Complete this table

Muscle	Action	Origin	Insertion	Nerve supply
Palmar interossei	(same as leg – palmar adduct, PAD)			
Dorsal interossei	(same as leg – dorsal abduct, DAB)			
Abductor digiti minimi				
Opponens digiti minimi				

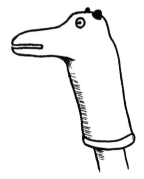

MEET 'LARRY THE LUMBRICAL'

The lumbricals flex the MCP joints and extend the PIPs rather like the position you would place your hand in when making a 'Larry the Lumbrical' glove puppet.

Larry the Lumbrical was thought up by Claire Cooper – with thanks.

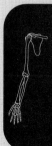

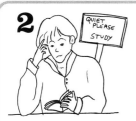

Judgement time

For all muscles of the upper limb you need to know:

- ❏ Origin
- ❏ Insertion
- ❏ Action
- ❏ Functional (applied) anatomy
- ❏ Nerve supply.

2

1 Write individual muscles' names on separate cards, randomly pick cards and make sure that you can describe origin, action, insertion and nerve supply for the muscle chosen.

2 For each muscle in the upper limb, think of a functional activity for which that muscle might be needed.

3 While you are watching your favourite TV programme analyse the muscle activity you can see in the living body.

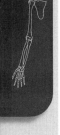

NERVES OF THE UPPER LIMB

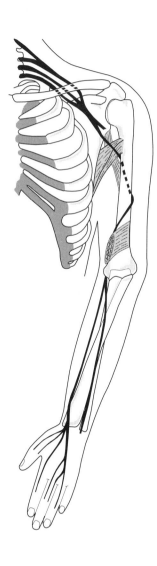

Nerves of the upper limb

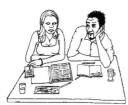

In this chapter you should be able to describe (written and orally):

1 Root level

2 Relations

3 Major branches

4 Innervations

5 Signs and symptoms resulting from lesions of the nerves listed below.

- ❏ Musculocutaneous nerve
- ❏ Axillary nerve
- ❏ Median nerve
- ❏ Ulnar nerve
- ❏ Radial nerve.

You need to know the dermatomes and myotomes of the lower and upper limbs.

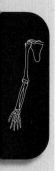

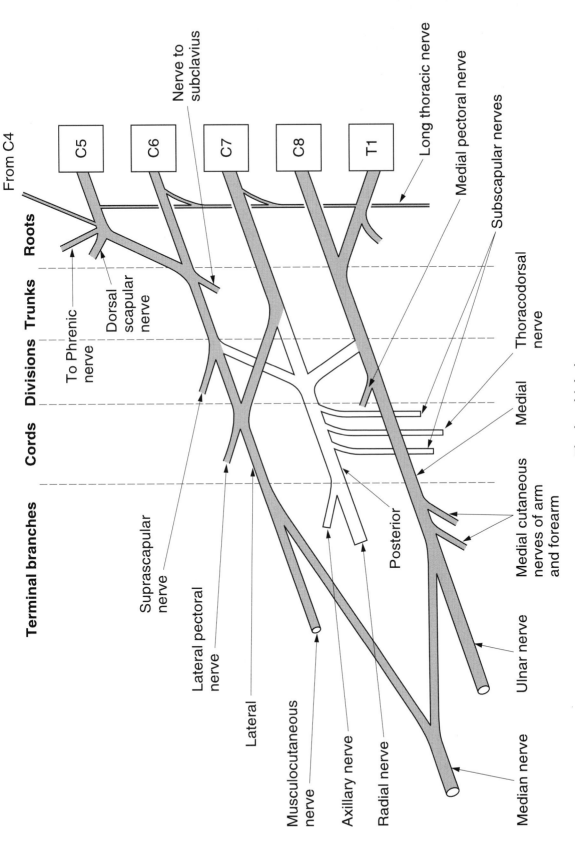

The brachial plexus.

Nerves of the upper limb

THE BRACHIAL PLEXUS

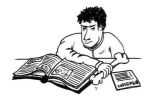

What is a plexus?

How can I remember the divisions of the plexus?

Really	_Roots_
Tight	_Trunks_
Denims	_Divisions_
Cause	_Cords_
Blotches	_Branches_

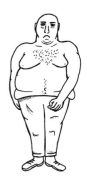

THE MUSCULOCUTANEOUS NERVE

(The BBC nerve!)

- Arises from lateral cord of brachial plexus C5, 6, 7
- Descends between axillary artery and coracobrachialis, which it pierces
- Then runs between biceps and coracobrachialis to reach lateral side of the arm
- Pierces deep fascia at the elbow as the lateral cutaneous nerve of the arm.

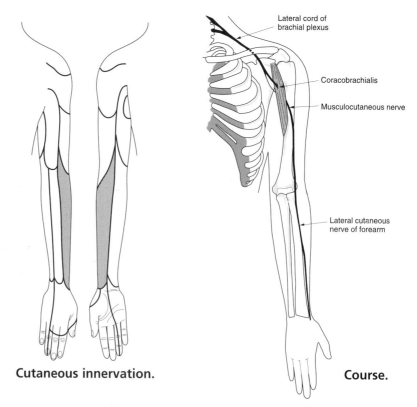

Lateral cord of brachial plexus

Coracobrachialis

Musculocutaneous nerve

Lateral cutaneous nerve of forearm

Cutaneous innervation.

Course.

The musculocutaneous nerve supplies Biceps, Brachialis and Coracobrachialis (remember BBC!).

THE AXILLARY NERVE

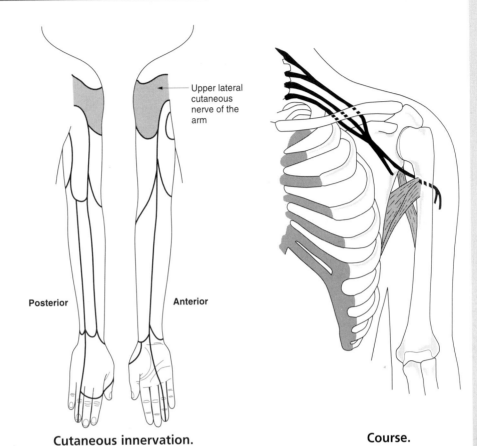

Upper lateral cutaneous nerve of the arm

Posterior   Anterior

Cutaneous innervation.

Course.

- Arises from posterior cord brachial plexus C5, 6
- Descends behind axillary artery in front of subscapularis
- Passes inferior to shoulder joint then through quadrangular space
- Supplies shoulder joint
- Splits into anterior and posterior branches
- Anterior branch winds round surgical neck of humerus to supply anterior deltoid
- Posteriorly is teres minor, posterior fibres are deltoid and it continues as lateral cutaneous nerve of the arm – supplies skin over lower deltoid and lateral triceps.

1 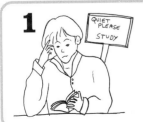 The axillary nerve may be injured in shoulder dislocations – which muscles would be paralysed if this were the case?

Nerves of the upper limb

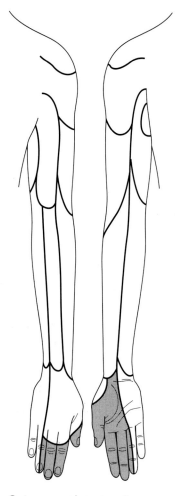

Cutaneous innervation.

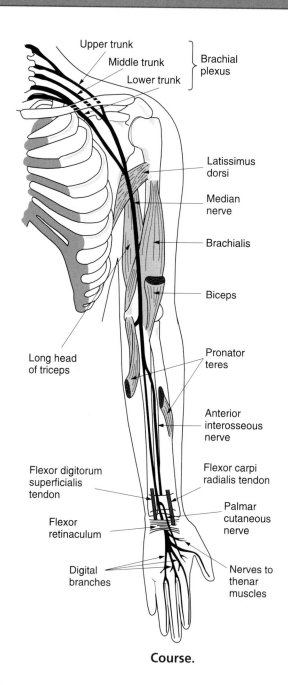

Course.

Upper trunk
Middle trunk
Lower trunk
Brachial plexus

Latissimus dorsi

Median nerve

Brachialis

Biceps

Pronator teres

Anterior interosseous nerve

Flexor carpi radialis tendon

Palmar cutaneous nerve

Nerves to thenar muscles

Long head of triceps

Flexor digitorum superficialis tendon

Flexor retinaculum

Digital branches

- Arises partly from lateral cord C5, 6, 7 partly from medial cord C8, T1 of brachial plexus
- Descends under biceps lateral to brachial artery then medially
- It lies on top of brachialis
- Then is crossed by the bicipital aponeurosis
- Enters the forearm between two heads of pronator teres
- Travels between flexor digitorum profundus and superficialis
- Becomes superficial at the wrist but deep to palmaris longus
- Passes through the carpal tunnel.

The median nerve sends articular branches to the elbow joint and supplies:

- Pronator teres
- Flexor carpi radialis
- Palmaris longus
- Flexor digitorum superficialis
- Flexor digitorum profundus
- Flexor pollicis longus
- Pronator quadratus.

Once through the carpal tunnel, the median nerve enters the hand and it divides into lateral and medial branches. The lateral branch supplies abductor pollicis brevis, flexor pollicis brevis, opponens pollicis and first lumbrical. The medial branch supplies the second lumbrical, and has many digital branches to nail beds, IP joints and MCP joints.

The median nerve may be injured by deep cuts. This gives loss of flexion of IP joints, except for the distal ones in ring and little fingers. MCPs can still be flexed by lumbricals and interossei. Thumb cannot oppose or abduct deformity (monkey hand). The thumb lies in same plane as hand, with wasting of the thenar eminence.

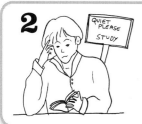

2 Compression in the carpal tunnel or carpal tunnel syndrome, affects the thenar muscles, lateral two lumbricals, and leads to sensory changes in the hand.

What can cause carpal tunnel syndrome?

THE RADIAL NERVE

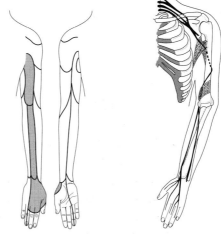

Cutaneous innervation.   Course.

- ☞ Posterior cord brachial plexus C5, 6, 7, 8 (T1)
- ☞ Passes anterior to subscapularis, latissimus dorsi, and teres major
- ☞ Enters spiral groove of humerus
- ☞ Pierces intermuscular septum to enter anterior compartment to lie between brachialis and brachioradialis
- ☞ In front of lateral humeral epicondyle, it splits into superficial and deep branches.

The radial nerve supplies mainly:

- ☞ Triceps, anconeus
- ☞ Brachioradialis
- ☞ ECRL, ECRB
- ☞ Supinator
- ☞ Long finger extensors
- ☞ Abductor pollicis longus
- ☞ Thumb extensors.

Injury to the radial nerve leads to an inability to extend wrist/fingers, with wrist drop. There is a loss of synergistic action of wrist extensors when making a fist (what does this statement mean?).

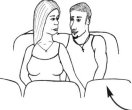

The radial nerve may be damaged by fracture to the humeral shaft where it winds round the bone – always check these fractures for signs of a wrist drop. It may be injured by axillary crutches used incorrectly.

What is a Saturday night palsy?

How do I remember what the radial nerve supplies?

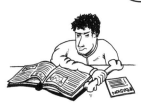

I would like to _extend_ a _radiant_ thank you for buying this book. (The _radial_ nerve predominantly supplies the _exten_sors of the arm.)

THE ULNAR NERVE

- ☞ Medial cord of the brachial plexus, C8 and T1
- ☞ Medial to axillary artery
- ☞ Travels anterior to triceps
- ☞ Pierces intermuscular septum distally in the arm to enter the posterior compartment of the arm
- ☞ Between medial humeral epicondyle and the olecranon, lying in the ulnar groove
- ☞ Enters anterior compartment lying between two heads of flexor carpi ulnaris (FCU)
- ☞ Descends forearm lying on flexor digitorum profundus (FDP) and is covered by FCU belly.

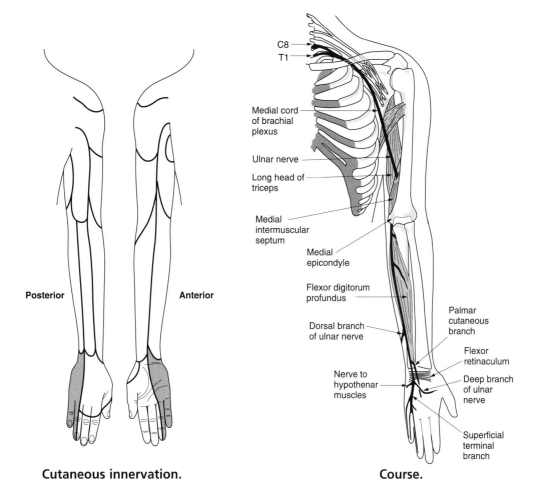

Cutaneous innervation.

Course.

Labels in figure: C8, T1, Medial cord of brachial plexus, Ulnar nerve, Long head of triceps, Medial intermuscular septum, Medial epicondyle, Flexor digitorum profundus, Dorsal branch of ulnar nerve, Nerve to hypothenar muscles, Palmar cutaneous branch, Flexor retinaculum, Deep branch of ulnar nerve, Superficial terminal branch, Posterior, Anterior

The ulnar nerve supplies:

- FCU
- Medial half of FDP
- Palmaris brevis
- Hypothenar muscles
- Medial two lumbricals
- Adductor pollicis
- Flexor pollicis brevis.

Sensory supply is to the palmar and dorsal aspect of little finger and half of ring fingers.

Injury to ulnar nerve (claw hand) leads to hyperextension of the 4/5th MCP joints and flexion of the IP joint. The little finger drifts into abduction and the hypothenar muscles atrophy.

Question: You bang your 'funny bone' on a chair. This sends pins and needles down the medial border of your forearm, your little finger and half of your ring finger also get pins and needles.

1 Which nerve have you hit?
2 Whereabouts have you compressed the nerve on its course?

3 What is paraesthesia?
4 What is anaesthesia?
5 What is hyperaesthesia?

Answers

☞ Ulnar nerve
☞ Posterior elbow between medial epicondyle and olecranon
☞ Abnormal sensation
☞ Absence of sensation
☞ Overly sensitive.

3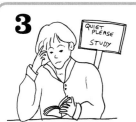

For each of the nerves in this chapter, make sure that you are able to describe the:

☞ Motor loss
☞ Sensory loss
☞ Functional loss
☞ Typical deformities

commonly resulting from paralysis of each nerve of the upper limb.

Make sure that you can demonstrate the dermatomes and myotomes of the upper limb.

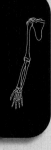

Draw the radial, median and ulnar nerves on these skeletons

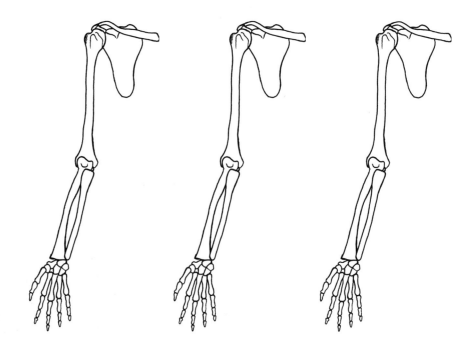

Dermatomes of the upper limb.

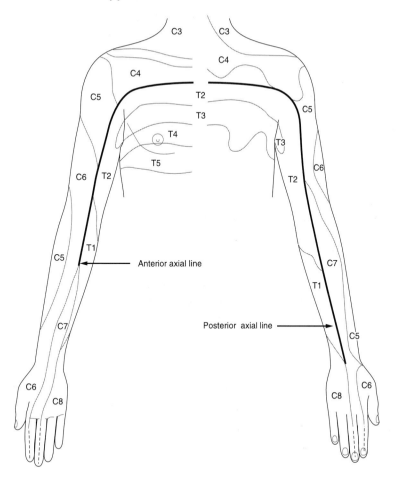

Draw the radial, median and ulnar nerves' sensory distribution on these arms

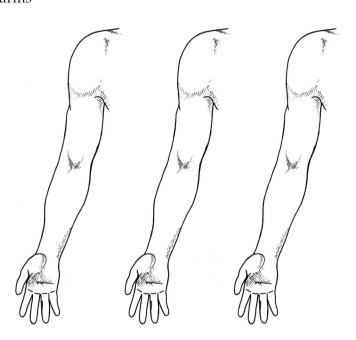

Nerves of the upper limb

Draw the dermatomes of the upper limb on this arm

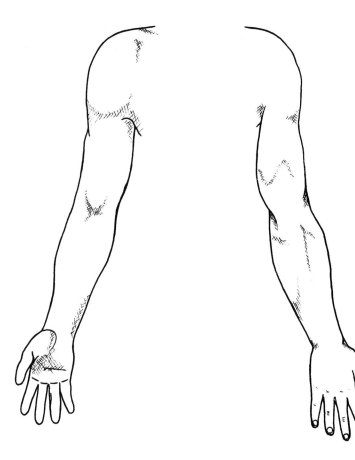

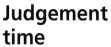

Judgement time

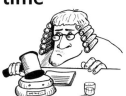

Can you describe (written and orally) for the nerves of the upper limb?

- ☞ root level
- ☞ relations
- ☞ major branches
- ☞ innervations
- ☞ signs and symptoms resulting from lesions of the nerves listed below.

  - ❑ musculocutaneous nerve
  - ❑ axillary nerve
  - ❑ median nerve
  - ❑ ulnar nerve
  - ❑ radial nerve.

- ☞ Do you know the dermatomes of the upper limb?

THE SPINE

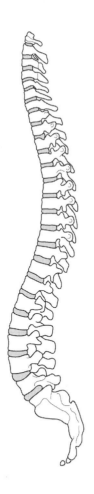

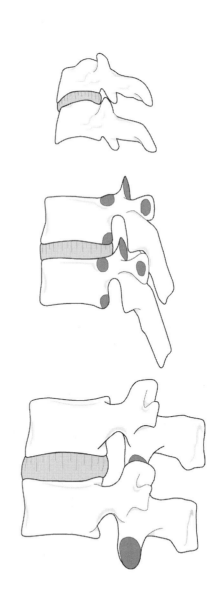

The spine

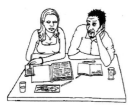

Upon completion of this chapter the self-directed study sessions and relevant lectures/tutorials, you should be able to:

1 Describe a typical cervical, thoracic and lumbar vertebra

2 Describe the structure and function of an intervertebral disc

3 Describe the structure and function of the sacroiliac joint

4 Describe the structure and function of the human spinal column

5 Describe the articulations of the human spine

6 Describe the following ligaments:

- ❑ Alar
- ❑ Transverse
- ❑ Ligamentum nuchae
- ❑ Ligamentum flavum
- ❑ Anterior longitudinal ligament
- ❑ Posterior longitudinal ligament
- ❑ Interspinous ligament
- ❑ Supraspinous ligament.

7 Have a knowledge of the major muscles acting on the spine.

OK here we go with one of the most complex and fascinating parts of the body . . .

   Medicine has worked hard to get to grips with the human spine. As long ago as the 17th century BC, an Egyptian papyrus described the difference between cervical sprain, fracture, and fracture–dislocation (Sanan & Rengachary 1996).

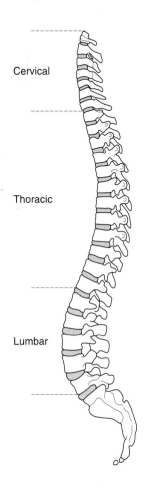

Cervical

Thoracic

Lumbar

THE BONES

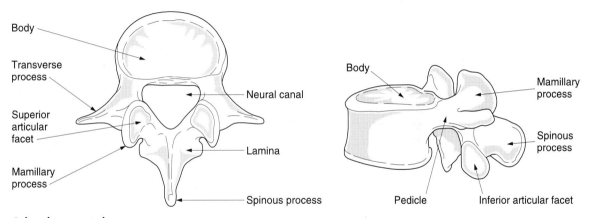

Body

Transverse process

Superior articular facet

Mamillary process

Neural canal

Lamina

Spinous process

Body

Mamillary process

Spinous process

Pedicle

Inferior articular facet

A lumbar vertebra.

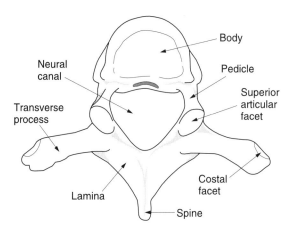

A thoracic vertebra.

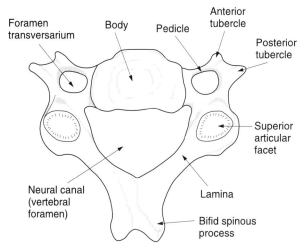

A cervical vertebra.

It would be a worthwhile exercise to make a summary of the similarities and differences between cervical, thoracic and lumbar vertebrae, including how each is specialised and why.

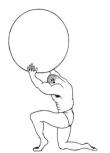

The atlas and the axis

These are the names given to the first and second cervical vertebrae.

Atlas = C1.

Atlas was the Greek God who it was believed supported the universe on his shoulders. In anatomical terms, the atlas supports the head.

Axis = C2.

These bones are not shaped like their other fellow vertebrae.

The atlas (C1).

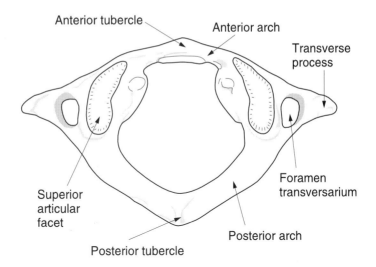

The axis (C2).

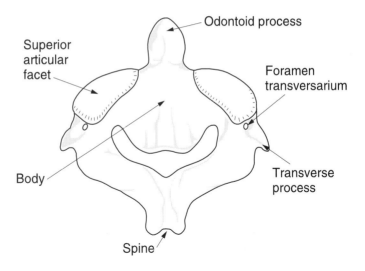

Look at this picture

☞ Can you now work out what travels though the holes in either side of the cervical vertebrae?

☞ Blockage or narrowing of the vertebral artery can lead to vertebrobasilar insufficiency (VBI); in other words lightheadedness or fainting upon certain neck movements. This is an important concept in examination and assessment of the spine.

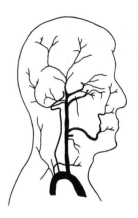

The spine

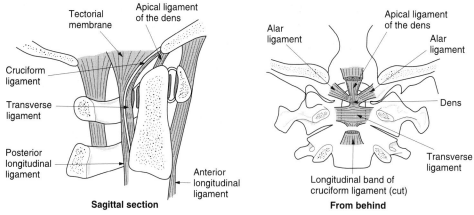

Sagittal section

- Tectorial membrane
- Apical ligament of the dens
- Cruciform ligament
- Transverse ligament
- Posterior longitudinal ligament
- Anterior longitudinal ligament

From behind

- Alar ligament
- Apical ligament of the dens
- Alar ligament
- Dens
- Transverse ligament
- Longitudinal band of cruciform ligament (cut)

Atlanto–axial articulation.

The alar ligaments basically join the odontoid to the skull. Think of them as the horns on a Viking's helmet!

THE STRUCTURE OF THE SPINE

The important thing about the human spine is that it is very flexible and also very stable. It achieves this by having many individual joints, each of which only moves a small amount, but add them all together and they form a mobile structure.

The motion segment.

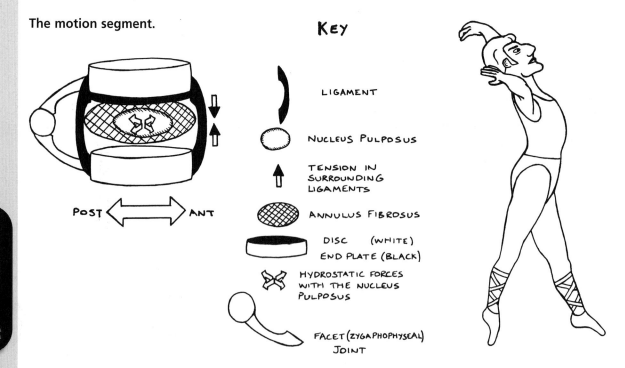

KEY

- LIGAMENT
- NUCLEUS PULPOSUS
- TENSION IN SURROUNDING LIGAMENTS
- ANNULUS FIBROSUS
- DISC (WHITE) END PLATE (BLACK)
- HYDROSTATIC FORCES WITH THE NUCLEUS PULPOSUS
- FACET (ZYGAPHOPHYSEAL) JOINT

POST ⟷ ANT

The spine allows support and movement of the skull, flexion of the neck and back, anchor sites for the ribs, and support and protection for the spinal cord. It consists of seven cervical vertebrae,

12 thoracic vertebrae, and five lumbar vertebrae. It ends inferiorly at the sacrum, a bone made of five fused vertebrae which anchors the spine to the pelvic girdle, and the coccyx. Between each vertebra is an intervertebral disc made of cartilage, which acts as a shock absorber, to cushion the vertebral column from trauma. The disc also maintains the stability of the spinal column and yet permits small movements between two adjacent vertebrae.

Intervertebral discs are like lecturers – they have a hard exterior and a soft squishy centre!

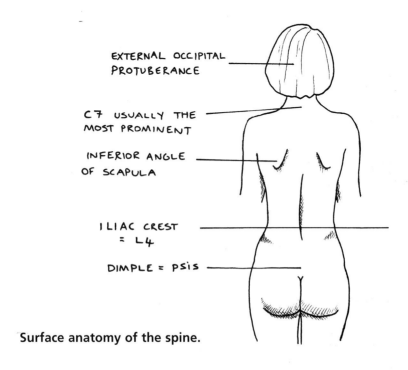

EXTERNAL OCCIPITAL PROTUBERANCE

C7 USUALLY THE MOST PROMINENT

INFERIOR ANGLE OF SCAPULA

ILIAC CREST = L4

DIMPLE = PSIS

Surface anatomy of the spine.

The motion segment (simplified)

Like a doughnut between two bricks, the disc has a vertebra above and below it. Together, these make up the so-called 'motion segment'.

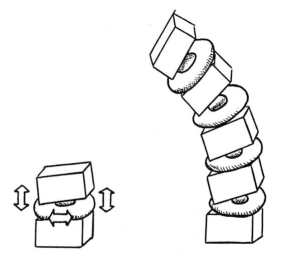

The soft-centred doughnut

The disc consists of an outer ring known as the annulus fibrosus and a gel-like portion called the nucleus pulposus. (The analogy to a jam doughnut works well). Intervertebral discs contain fibrocytes and chondrocytes in elaborate avascular matrices of collagen and proteoglycans (Guiot and Fessler 2000). The resulting column is remarkably stable and mobile in equal proportions. The disc is pre-stressed by tension in the surrounding ligaments and the nucleus acts hydrostatically during loading. The intervertebral discs tend to become thicker as you descend the spinal column, and they tend to be wedge shaped. The combined effect of these multiple wedges is to give the spine its three curvatures when viewed laterally. The curvatures in the cervical, lumbar and thoracic spine add to the strength of the spine and its ability to withstand compression; this also means that the line of gravity weaves anterior and posterior to the discs. The normal disc is remarkably strong and resilient to compressive loading and twisting movements, to the extent that falls from a height will often cause fracture of the vertebral body itself rather than damage to the disc.

The intervertebral disc.

Key	Comments
E = end plates	❑ Permit osmosis ❑ Protect the vertebra from pressure ❑ Anchor the disc
N = nucleus pulposus	❑ Type 11 collagen only ❑ Hydrophilic ❑ Kept in check by the annulus
A = annulus fibrosus	❑ Type 1 collagen (typical of tendon) provides the disc with tensile strength ❑ Type 11 collagen (typical of cartilage) provides the disc with compressive strength

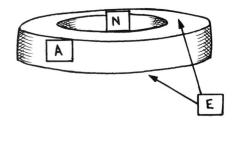

The inelastic envelope provided by the annulus fibrosus (the fibres of which have a criss-cross arrangement of collagen bundles) restrains the nucleus. It has been known for some time that the outer portion of the annulus possesses nerve endings mainly in the outer (lateral) half of the annulus fibrosus, and hence may produce pain (Yoshizawa *et al.* 1980). This may explain the presence of back symptoms which occur even when discs appear intact and normal (Bogduk 1991).

Above and below each disc is the end plate. This has several functions: it permits osmosis from the vertebral body both in and out of the disc, it restrains the disc and it may protect the vertebrae from pressure.

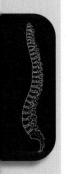

It can be difficult to visualise how things are put together in the spine, so try this exercise. Make your own 'tasty' spinal column. This spinal column can only help you to lose weight as part of a calorie-controlled diet.

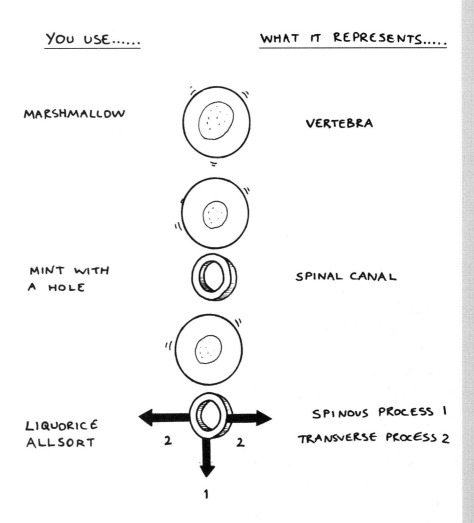

YOU USE......

MARSHMALLOW — VERTEBRA

MINT WITH A HOLE — SPINAL CANAL

WHAT IT REPRESENTS.....

LIQUORICE ALLSORT — SPINOUS PROCESS 1 / TRANSVERSE PROCESS 2

2 2

1

In this analogy, the disc sits on top and underneath each marshmallow, the spinal cord runs through the polo mint. Compare your finished model to the diagrams in the book, and make sure you understand and can name the parts of the vertebra, then eat your model.

The facet joints

The orientation of the facet joints controls the direction and amount of movement possible in the spine. For example, in the thoracic spine, they are aligned in such a way as to permit free rotation.

The spine

This is not the case in the lumbar spine where they are arranged so as to limit rotation. See the diagrams below.

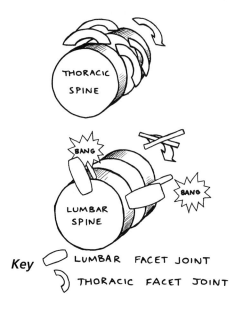

The facet joints (zygapophyseal) joints)

- 🖎 How are facet joints arranged in the cervical spine?
- 🖎 What are they?
- 🖎 Where are they?
- 🖎 What is their function?

The uncovertebral joints

- 🖎 What are they?
- 🖎 Where are they?
- 🖎 What is their function?

The ligaments of the spine

- 🖎 Anterior longitudinal ligament (1 below)
- 🖎 Posterior longitudinal ligament (3 below)
- 🖎 Intertransverse ligament (2 below)
- 🖎 Interspinous ligament (4 below)
- 🖎 Supraspinous ligament (5 below)
- 🖎 Ligamentum nuchae (self-directed)
- 🖎 Ligamentum flavum (self-directed).

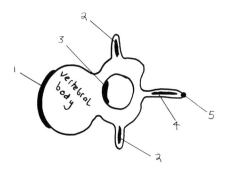

Diagram of a vertebra from above.

For each of the ligaments on this diagram complete the table

Ligament	Attachments	Function
Supraspinous		
Anterior longitudinal		
Posterior longitudinal		
Interspinous		
Ligamentum flavum		

THE MUSCLES OF THE SPINE

The abdominal muscles

- Rectus abdominis
- Internal oblique
- External oblique
- Transversus abdominis.

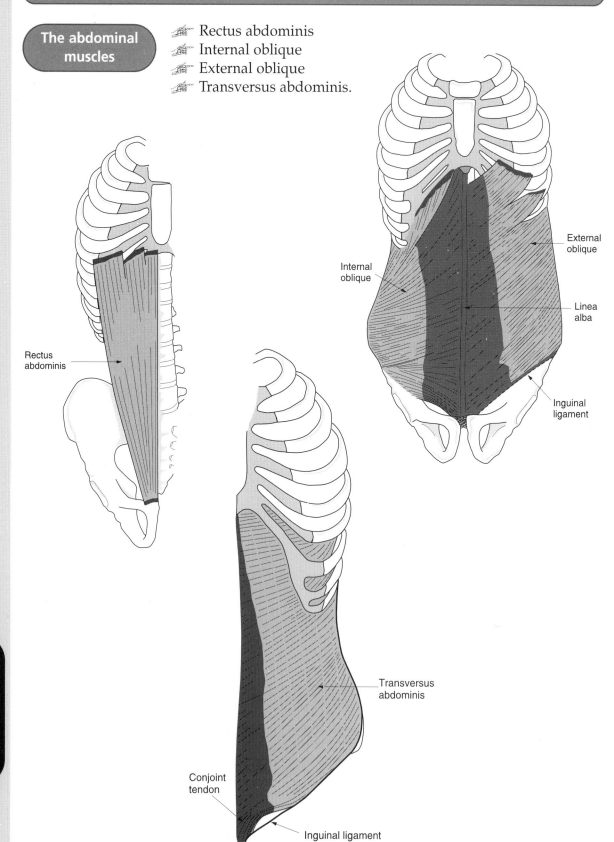

Rectus abdominis

External oblique

Internal oblique

Linea alba

Inguinal ligament

Transversus abdominis

Conjoint tendon

Inguinal ligament

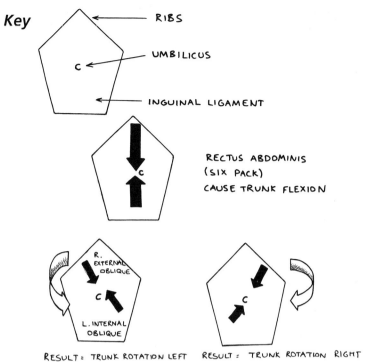

Key

RIBS

UMBILICUS

C

INGUINAL LIGAMENT

RECTUS ABDOMINIS
(SIX PACK)
CAUSE TRUNK FLEXION

R. EXTERNAL OBLIQUE

L. INTERNAL OBLIQUE

RESULT: TRUNK ROTATION LEFT   RESULT: TRUNK ROTATION RIGHT

WHEN THE INTERNAL
AND EXTERNAL
OBLIQUES ON THE
SAME SIDE WORK
TOGETHER, THE NET
RESULT IS SIDE
FLEXION TO THAT
SIDE.

Muscles flexing the trunk

Complete this table

Name	Origin	Insertion	Action	Function
Rectus abdominis				
External oblique				

The spine

Name	Origin	Insertion	Action	Function
Internal oblique				
Psoas major/minor				

Muscles extending the trunk

Complete this table

Name	Origin	Insertion	Action	Function
Quadratus lumborum				
Multifidus				
Semispinalis				
Erector spinae				

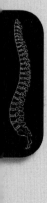

Erector spinae

This is a complex of muscles which has origins on the sacrum and lumbar spine.

It passes upwards and splits into three bundles:

☞ Iliocostalis
☞ Spinalis
☞ Longissumus.

What does it do?

☞ It extends the trunk
☞ It resists flexion
☞ It helps maintain the lordosis.

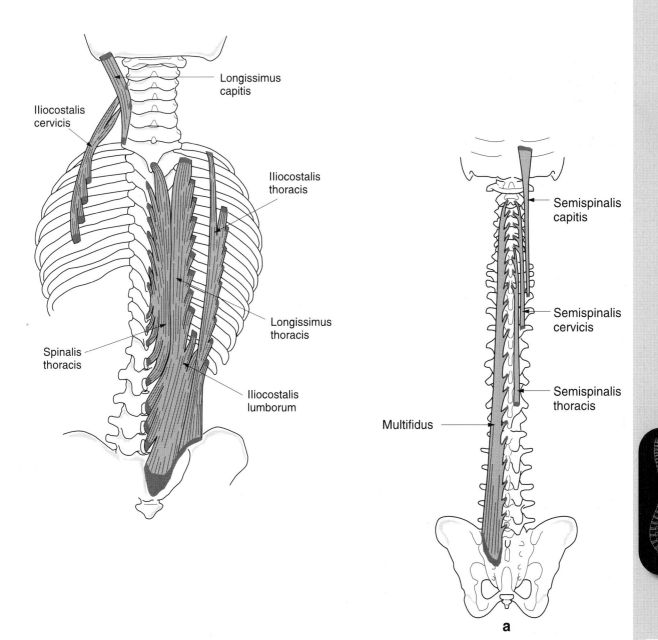

Longissimus capitis

Iliocostalis cervicis

Iliocostalis thoracis

Longissimus thoracis

Spinalis thoracis

Iliocostalis lumborum

Semispinalis capitis

Semispinalis cervicis

Semispinalis thoracis

Multifidus

a

THE INTERVERTEBRAL DISC AND ITS PATHOLOGY

A normal intervertebral disc is crucial if normal motion of the human spine is to occur (Thompson *et al.* 2000).

Think of the disc in this way.

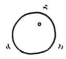

The discs of a baby are like squash balls.

The discs of an adult are like jam doughnuts, soft centred with a hard outside.

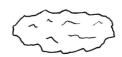

The disc of an 80-year-old is like a popadum, dry and brittle.

Intervertebral disc pathology

A normal disc has a hard outer rim called an annulus and a soft pulpy or gel-like centre called a nucleus.

STRUCTURE

The disc is normally hydrophilic (water-loving). You are taller when you wake up in the morning because the disc absorbs water overnight as you lie down. With age it becomes less hydrophilic and loses height as it desiccates (dries out).

Discs get thicker as one descends the column (they have to carry more weight) and they help to contribute towards the spinal curves.

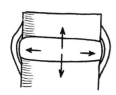

In a normal disc, stresses and strains are evenly distributed throughout the disc. The disc is so strong that a fall from a height will often fracture the vertebra itself rather than burst the disc. Healthy discs are water loving (hydrophilic) and swell, pushing adjacent vertebrae apart, tightening surrounding ligaments.

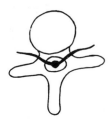

The disc lies in close proximity to the spinal cord, nerve roots and intervertebral foramina.

The function of the discs is to give each segment stability with a small degree of mobility. When all the spinal column movements are added together, the spine is very mobile but retains its stability.

The intervertebral disc and its pathology

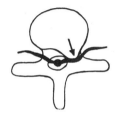

Repeated flexed postures or trauma places massive stress on the posterior of the disc, this may cause the nucleus to herniate or bulge, like the jam leaking out of a jam doughnut. Sometimes a piece of disc breaks off and floats around. This is sequestration.

Schmorl's nodes

Occasionally, the disc herniates through the end plate itself. This is called a Schmorl's node.

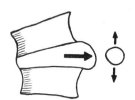

Schmorl's node.

Prolapsed inter-vertebral disc (PID)

Because of the anatomy of surrounding ligaments, most protrusions are posterolateral (back and to one side). The significance of this is that the adjacent nerve root may become inflamed or 'trapped'. This will result in referred pain in the distribution of the corresponding nerve supply. A large or central bulge may cause spinal cord compression, and so-called long tract signs such as loss of bowel and bladder control and spasticity.

Lumbar spondylosis (disc degeneration or wear and tear)

Along with prolapse, this is probably the most common spinal condition. The disc loses height with age. It is less good at taking stresses and strains and spinal movement diminishes. Because of this loss of joint space, more strain is put on the facet joints, causing them to degenerate.

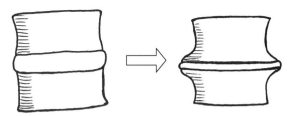

PROFESSOR ASKS

If the disc itself has virtually no nerve supply, why should a prolapsed intervertebral disc give a patient so much pain?

Clues:

Think about the surrounding structures.

Think about the by-products of the inflammatory process.

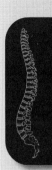

221

☞ Why are anterior protrusions relatively asymptomatic?

Clue: what structures are anterior in the spinal column?

☞ Why are most protrusions in a posterolateral direction, as the one shown above?

Clue: which ligament lies posterior to the disc and would therefore tend to resist posterior disc displacement?

THE SACROILIAC JOINT

☞ Where is it? It is an L-shaped joint between the ilium and the ala of the sacrum roughly marked out as a line from the posterior superior iliac spine (PSIS) running 25° superolaterally to inferomedially 2.5 cm either way from the PSIS.

☞ How is it classified? The weird thing is that it is partly synovial and partly fibrous.

☞ The main ligaments are anterior and posterior.

☞ How much movement occurs at this joint? Depends who you ask! Wang and Dumas (1998) did studies on cadavers and claim that 'Lateral rotation and nutation rotation of the sacrum were found to be the predominant motion, though the values were limited to less than 1.2°. Both the anterior and posterior sacroiliac ligaments were found to play an important role in resisting rotations at the joints.'

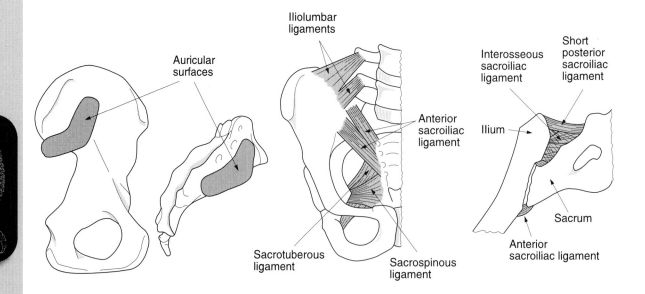

The sacroiliac joint.

DEGENERATIVE SPINAL DISORDERS AT A GLANCE

Your notes

Normal spine

Spondylosis

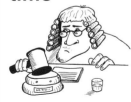

Spondylolisthesis

Judgement time

Can you:

1 Describe a typical cervical, thoracic and lumbar vertebra?
2 Describe the structure and function of an intervertebral disc?
3 Describe the structure and function of the sacroiliac joint?
4 Describe the structure and function of the human spinal column?
5 Describe the articulations of the human spine?
6 Describe these ligaments?

  ❑ Alar
  ❑ Transverse
  ❑ Ligamentum nuchae
  ❑ Ligamentum flavum
  ❑ Anterior longitudinal ligament
  ❑ Posterior longitudinal ligament
  ❑ Interspinous ligament
  ❑ Supraspinous ligament.

7 Do you have knowledge of the major muscles acting on the spine?

ANATOMY PRE-EXAM CHECKLIST

LOWER LIMB

Can you tick these boxes with confidence? If you cannot, make sure you can do so before your exams (written and practical).

Can I . . .

	Pelvis	Femur	Patella	Tibia	Fibula	All the bones of the foot
Describe in detail these bones						
Be able to palpate all major bony landmarks						
Know the functions of the skeleton & various types of bone						

	Hip	Knee	Patello-femoral	Superior tibiofibular	Inferior tibiofibular	Ankle	Subtalar	Small joints of the foot
Classify these joints								
Describe movements occurring at each joint and limiting factors for each								
Be able to relate the structure of the joint to its function								

	Hip joint	Knee joint	Patellofemoral joint	Ankle joint	Subtalar joint	Small joints of the foot
Talk to an examiner in *detail* for five minutes about						
Describe the common features of each joints						

	Origin	Insertion	Action	Nerve supply	Applied/functional anatomy
For *every* muscle of the lower limb, do you know the . . .					

For the following nerves, can you describe in written detail	Write in detail for exams
Sciatic nerve	
Tibial nerve	
Common peroneal nerve	
Deep peroneal nerve	
Superficial peroneal nerve	
Obturator nerve (main branches only)	
Femoral nerve (main branches only)	

Appendix

Can you tick these boxes with confidence? If you cannot, make sure you can do so before your exams (written and practical).

Can I . . .

	Scapula	Clavicle	Humerus	Radius	Ulna	All the bones of the hand
Describe in detail these bones						
Be able to palpate all major bony landmarks						

	SCJ	ACJ	Glenohumeral	Subacromial	Elbow	Radio-ulnar	Wrist	Hand
Classify these joints								
Describe movements occurring at each joint and limiting factors for each								
Be able to relate the structure of the joint to its function								

Talk to an examiner in detail for five minutes about						
Describe the common features of these joints						

	Origin	Insertion	Action	Nerve supply	Applied/functional anatomy
For every muscle of the upper limb, do you know the . . .					

For the following nerves, can you describe in written detail	Write in detail for exams
Radial	
Ulnar	
Musculocutaneous	
Median	
Axillary	

BIBLIOGRAPHY

Aagaard, H. and Verdonk, R. (1999). Function of the normal meniscus and consequences of meniscal resection. *Scand J Med Sci Sports* **9**(3): 134–40.

Adams, M. A., Freeman, B. J. *et al.* (2000). Mechanical initiation of intervertebral disc degeneration. *Spine* **25**(13): 1625–36.

Ahmad, I. (1975). Articular muscle of the knee – articularis genus. *Bull Hosp Joint Dis* **36**(1): 58–60.

Andrews, J. R., Carson, W. G., Jr. *et al.* (1985). Glenoid labrum tears related to the long head of the biceps. *Am J Sports Med* **13**(5): 337–41.

Bagg, S. D. and Forrest, W. J. (1988). A biomechanical analysis of scapular rotation during arm abduction in the scapular plane. *Am J Phys Med Rehabil* **67**(6): 238–45.

Bogduk, N., Johnson, G. *et al.* (1998). The morphology and biomechanics of latissimus dorsi. *Clin Biomech (Bristol, Avon)* **13**(6): 377–85.

Cober, S. R. and Trumble, T. E. (2001). Arthroscopic repair of triangular fibrocartilage complex injuries. *Orthop Clin North Am* **32**(2): 279–94, viii.

Dolan, P. and Adams, M. A. (1998). Repetitive lifting tasks fatigue the back muscles and increase the bending moment acting on the lumbar spine. *J Biomech* **31**(8): 713–21.

Englund, M., Roos, E. M. *et al.* (2001). Patient-relevant outcomes fourteen years after meniscectomy: influence of type of meniscal tear and size of resection. *Rheumatology (Oxford)* **40**(6): 631–9.

Fischer-Rasmussen, T. and Jensen, P. E. (2000). Proprioceptive sensitivity and performance in anterior cruciate ligament-deficient knee joints. *Scand J Med Sci Sports* **10**(2): 85–9.

Giddings, V. L., Beaupre, G. S. *et al.* (2000). Calcaneal loading during walking and running. *Med Sci Sports Exerc* **32**(3): 627–34.

Goto, H., Shuler, F. D. *et al.* (2000). Gene therapy for meniscal injury: enhanced synthesis of proteoglycan and collagen by meniscal cells transduced with a TGFbeta(1)gene. *Osteoarthritis Cartilage* **8**(4): 266–71.

Guiot, B. H. and Fessler, R. G. (2000). Molecular biology of degenerative disc disease. *Neurosurgery* **47**(5): 1034–40.

Hunt, A. E., Smith, R. M. *et al.* (2001). Extrinsic muscle activity, foot motion and ankle joint moments during the stance phase of walking. *Foot Ankle Int* **22**(1): 31–41.

Jobe, C. M. (1996). Superior glenoid impingement. Current concepts. *Clin Orthop* **330**: 98–107.

Kido, T., Itoi, E. *et al.* (2000). The depressor function of biceps on the head of the humerus in shoulders with tears of the rotator cuff. *J Bone Joint Surg Br* **82**(3): 416–19.

Makris, C. A., Georgoulis, A. D. *et al.* (2000). Posterior cruciate ligament architecture: evaluation under microsurgical dissection. *Arthroscopy* **16**(6): 627–32.

Michiels, I. and Grevenstein, J. (1995). Kinematics of shoulder abduction in the scapular plane. On the influence of abduction velocity and external load. *Clin Biomech (Bristol, Avon)* **10**(3): 137–43.

Nadler, S. F., Malanga, G. A. *et al.* (2001). Relationship between hip muscle imbalance and occurrence of low back pain in collegiate athletes: a prospective study. *Am J Phys Med Rehabil* **80**(8): 572–7.

Rodeo, S. A. (2001). Meniscal allografts – where do we stand? *Am J Sports Med* **29**(2): 246–61.

Sanan, A. and Rengachary, S. S. (1996). The history of spinal biomechanics. *Neurosurgery* **39**(4): 657–68; discussion 668–9.

Santaguida, P. L. and McGill, S. M. (1995). The psoas major muscle: a three-dimensional geometric study. *J Biomech* **28**(3): 339–45.

Self, B. P., Harris, S. *et al.* (2000). Ankle biomechanics during impact landings on uneven surfaces. *Foot Ankle Int* **21**(2): 138–44.

Simunic, D. I., Broom, N. D. *et al.* (2001). Biomechanical factors influencing nuclear disruption of the intervertebral disc. *Spine* **26**(11): 1223–30.

Swanepoel, M. W., Adams, L. M. *et al.* (1995). Human lumbar apophyseal joint damage and intervertebral disc degeneration. *Ann Rheum Dis* **54**(3): 182–8.

Thompson, R. E., Pearcy, M. J. *et al.* (2000). Disc lesions and the mechanics of the intervertebral joint complex. *Spine* **25**(23): 3026–35.

Wang, M. and Dumas, G. A. (1998). Mechanical behavior of the female sacroiliac joint and influence of the anterior and posterior sacroiliac ligaments under sagittal loads. *Clin Biomech (Bristol, Avon)* **13**(4–5): 293–9.

Yoshizawa, H., O'Brien, J. P. *et al.* (1980). The neuropathology of intervertebral discs removed for low-back pain. *J Pathol* **132**(2): 95–104.